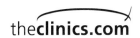

theclinics.com

OTOLARYNGOLOGIC CLINICS
OF NORTH AMERICA

ENT Emergencies

GUEST EDITORS
John L. Dornhoffer, MD
Rakesh K. Chandra, MD

June 2008 • Volume 41 • Number 3

SAUNDERS

An Imprint of Elsevier, Inc.
PHILADELPHIA   LONDON   TORONTO   MONTREAL   SYDNEY   TOKYO

W.B. SAUNDERS COMPANY
A Division of Elsevier Inc.

1600 John F. Kennedy Boulevard, Suite 1800, Philadelphia, PA 19103–2899

http://www.theclinics.com

OTOLARYNGOLOGIC CLINICS	**Volume 41, Number 3**
OF NORTH AMERICA	**ISSN 0030–6665**
June 2008	**ISBN-13: 978-1-4160-5829-8**
Editor: Joanne Husovski	**ISBN-10: 1-4160-5829-X**

Otolaryngologic Clinics of North America (ISSN 0030–6665) is published bimonthly by Elsevier Inc., 360 Park Avenue South, New York, NY 10010-1710. Months of issue are February, April, June, August, October, and December. Business and Editorial Offices: 1600 John F. Kennedy Blvd., Suite 1800, Philadelphia, PA 19103-2899. Customer Service Office: 6277 Sea Harbor Drive, Orlando, FL 32887-4800. Periodicals postage paid at New York, NY and additional mailing offices. Subscription price is $240.00 per year (US individuals), $448.00 per year (US institutions), $117.00 per year (US student/resident), $315.00 per year (Canadian individuals), $550.00 per year (Canadian institutions), $333.00 per year (international individuals), $550.00 per year (international institutions), $170.00 per year (international & Canadian student/resident). Foreign air speed delivery is included in all *Clinics'* subscription prices. All prices are subject to change without notice. **POSTMASTER:** Send address changes to *Otolaryngologic Clinics of North America*, Elsevier Periodicals Customer Service, 6277 Sea Harbor Drive, Orlando, FL 32887-4800. **Customer Service: 1-800-654-2452 (US). From outside the United States, call 1-407-563-6020. Fax: 1-407-563-8521. E-mail: JournalsCustomerService-usa@elsevier.com.**

Otolaryngologic Clinics of North America is also published in Spanish by McGraw-Hill Interamericana Editores S.A., P.O. Box 5-237, 06500 Mexico D.F., Mexico.

Otolaryngologic Clinics of North America is covered in *Index Medicus, Current Contents/Clinical Medicine, Excerpta Medica, BIOSIS, Science Citation Index*, and *ISI/BIOMED*.

Printed in the United States of America.

GUEST EDITORS

JOHN L. DORNHOFFER, MD, Professor and Director, Division of Neurotology, Department Otolaryngology/Head and Neck Surgery, University of Arkansas for Medical Sciences; Medical Director, ENT Clinic and Audiology Services, University of Arkansas for Medical Sciences; and Professor, Department of Neurobiology and Developmental Sciences, University of Arkansas for Medical Sciences, Little Rock, AK, USA

RAKESH K. CHANDRA, MD, Division of Nasal and Sinus Disorders, Department of Otolaryngology-Head & Neck Surgery, University of Tennessee, Memphis, Tennessee

CONTRIBUTORS

SHAWN M. ALLEN, MD, University of Tennessee College of Medicine, Tennessee

MATTHEW J. CARFRAE, MD, Fellow, Department of Otolaryngology – Head and Neck Surgery, Division of Otology-Neurotology, University of Virginia Health System, Charlottesville, Virginia

CHRISTOPHER J. DANNER, MD, Tampa Bay Hearing and Balance Center, Otology/Neurotology/Skull Base Surgery, Harbourside Medical Tower, Tampa, Florida

G. PAUL DIGOY, MD, Assistant Professor of Otorhinolaryngology, Department of Otorhinolaryngology, University of Oklahoma; and Director of Pediatric Otorhinolaryngology, University of Oklahoma Medical Center, Oklahoma City, Oklahoma

VICTORIA A. EPSTEIN, MD, Resident Physician, Department of Otolaryngology – Head and Neck Surgery, Feinberg School of Medicine, Northwestern University, Chicago, Illinois

THOMAS O. GIFFORD, MD, Capt, MC, USAF, Resident, Division of Otolaryngology – Head and Neck Surgery, University of Utah School of Medicine, Salt Lake City, Utah

DAVID S. HAYNES, MD, Director, Division of Otology and Neurotology, The Otology Group of Vanderbilt, Vanderbilt University Medical Center, Nashville, Tennessee

FREEDOM JOHNSON, MD, Chief Resident, Department of Otolaryngology – Head and Neck Surgery, Case Western Reserve University, University Hospitals of Cleveland, Cleveland, Ohio

ROBERT C. KERN, MD, Professor and Chairman, Department of Otolaryngology – Head and Neck Surgery, Feinberg School of Medicine, Northwestern University, Chicago, Illinois

BRADLEY W. KESSER, MD, Assistant Professor, Department of Otolaryngology – Head and Neck Surgery, Division of Otology-Neurotology, University of Virginia Health System, Charlottesville, Virginia

BENJAMIN D. LIESS, MD, Resident, Department of Otolaryngology Head and Neck Surgery, University of Missouri–Columbia School of Medicine, Columbia, Missouri

CLIFF A. MEGERIAN, MD, FACS, Professor and Vice-Chairman, Otology & Neurotology, and Cochlear Implant Program, Department of Otolaryngology – Head and Neck Surgery, Case Western Reserve University, University Hospitals of Cleveland, Cleveland, Ohio

MATTHEW R. O'MALLEY, MD, The Otology Group Vanderbilt, Vanderbilt University, Nashville, Tennessee

RICHARD R. ORLANDI, MD, FACS, Associate Professor, Division of Otolaryngology – Head and Neck Surgery, University of Utah School of Medicine; Center for Therapeutic Biomaterials, University of Utah School of Medicine; and George E. Wahlen Veterans Affairs Medical Center, Salt Lake City, Utah

JAMES N. PALMER, MD, Associate Professor, Department of Otorhinolaryngology, Division of Rhinology, University of Pennsylvania Health System, Philadelphia, Pennsylvania

TROY D. SCHEIDT, MD, Assistant Professor, Department of Otolaryngology Head and Neck Surgery, University of Missouri–Columbia School of Medicine, Columbia, Missouri

MAROUN T. SEMAAN, MD, Clinical Fellow, House Ear Institute, Los Angeles, California

STEVEN E. SOBOL, MD, MSc, Director of Pediatric Otolaryngology, Department of Otolaryngology–Head and Neck Surgery, Emory University School of Medicine; and Chief, Children's Healthcare of Atlanta at Egleston, Atlanta, Georgia

ROSE MARY S. STOCKS, MD, Professor, Department of Otolaryngology – Head and Neck Surgery, University of Tennessee Health Science Center, Memphis, Tennessee

JERRY W. TEMPLER, MD, Professor, Department of Otolaryngology Head and Neck Surgery, University of Missouri–Columbia School of Medicine, Columbia, Missouri

JEROME W. THOMPSON, MD, MBA, Chairman and Professor, Department of Otolaryngology – Head and Neck Surgery, University of Tennessee Health Science Center, Memphis, Tennessee

FRANCISCO VIEIRA, MD, Assistant Professor, Department of Otolaryngology – Head and Neck Surgery, University of Tennessee Health Science Center; and Chief of Otolaryngology-Head and Neck Surgery, Regional Medical Center at Memphis-The Med Hospital, Memphis, Tennessee

KEVIN C. WELCH, MD, Fellow, Department of Otorhinolaryngology, Division of Rhinology, University of Pennsylvania Health System, Philadelphia, Pennsylvania

SYBONEY ZAPATA, MD, Assistant Professor, Department of Otolaryngology–Head and Neck Surgery, Emory University School of Medicine, Atlanta, Georgia

CONTENTS

> Deep neck infections present significant morbidity and mortality,
> particularly when associated with predisposing factors that impair
> a functional immunologic response. Familiarity with deep neck
> spaces and fascial planes is critical, because these form the basis for
> the emergent nature of the disease process. Common and
> potentially life-threatening complications include airway obstruc-
> tion, jugular vein thrombosis, descending mediastinitis, sepsis,
> acute respiratory distress syndrome, and disseminated intra-
> vascular coagulation. The most common primary sources of deep
> neck infection are odontogenic, tonsillar, salivary gland, foreign
> body, and malignancy. Microbiology typically reveals mixed
> bacterial flora, including anaerobic species, that can rapidly
> progress to a fulminating necrotizing fasciitis. The treatment
> cornerstone remains securing the airway, providing efficient
> drainage and appropriate antibiotics, and improving immunologic
> status. A prolonged hospital stay should be anticipated.

> Although often listed together in review articles and case series,
> tracheobronchial and esophageal foreign bodies can be dissimilar.

Airway foreign bodies can range widely in the severity of presentation. When to proceed with a diagnostic bronchoscopy is not always obvious and is based on three diagnostic tools: clinical history, physical examination, and radiography. Radiography plays a more central role in the diagnosis of an esophageal foreign body. In either condition, a delay in diagnosis leads to a greater complication rate. This article provides diagnostic and treatment guidelines in the management of aerodigestive foreign bodies.

Acute fulminant invasive fungal sinusitis in an immunocompromised host and bacterial rhinosinusitis with intracranial or orbital extension are challenging to manage and constitute true otolaryngic emergencies. In the absence of rapid diagnosis and treatment, these diseases can be fatal. In this article, the complications of bacterial rhinosinusitis are divided into three categories: local, orbital, and intracranial. They vary in their characteristics and severity according to their location, duration, and specific symptoms. This article reviews the pathophysiology, clinical presentation, diagnosis, and treatment options of acute invasive fungal sinusitis rhinosinusitis, the most common subtype in the United States.

Epistaxis is a common occurrence. The estimated lifetime incidence of epistaxis is approximately 60% and it ranges in severity from a minor nuisance to a life-threatening hemorrhage. Evaluation of recurrent or severe cases includes a search for underlying causes, such as bleeding disorders and neoplasia. Many techniques, materials, and procedures treat nasal bleeding effectively and sometimes more than one treatment must be used. Otolaryngologists must be prepared to deal with severe or refractory bleeding through the use of medications, packing materials, and radiologic or surgical interventions. This article reviews nasal vascular anatomy, common causes of epistaxis, and treatments, including biomaterials and minimally invasive surgical techniques.

Malignant otitis externa is an invasive, potentially life-threatening infection of the external ear and skull base that requires urgent diagnosis and treatment. It affects immunocompromised individuals, particularly those who have diabetes. The most common causative agent remains Pseudomonas aeruginosa. Definitive diagnosis is frequently elusive, requiring a high index of suspicion, various laboratory and imaging modalities, and histologic exclusion of malignancy. Long-term oral antipseudomonal agents have proven effective; however, pseudomonal antibiotic resistance patterns have emerged and therefore other bacterial and fungal causative agents must be considered. Adjunctive therapies, such as aggressive debridement and hyperbaric oxygen therapy, are reserved for extensive or unresponsive cases.

Infections of the upper airways are a frequent cause of morbidity in children. Viral laryngotracheobronchitis (croup) is the most common cause of stridor in children and usually has a self-limited course with occasional relapses in early childhood. Epiglottitis has become rare in developed countries with the advent of universal vaccinations against *Haemophilus influenzae*. It can be rapidly fatal, however, if not promptly recognized and appropriately managed. This article reviews the pathogenesis, epidemiology, clinical presentation, diagnosis, and management of these pediatric upper airway infections.

Securing the airway in a dyspneic patient is a challenging task because of the myriad causes and presentations. Initial assessment may demonstrate factors indicative of upper airway abnormalities; however, they may not be specific nor sensitive enough to accurately predict difficult intubation. A well-equipped airway cart must be immediately available. A standardized escalating approach to secure the airway in a difficult situation begins with a rapid sequence of attempts at standard intubation, followed by attempted tube introduction over a bougie or using a flexible endoscope or laryngeal mask, and finally surgical interventions including cricothyrotomy or tracheotomy.

Among the several risks encountered in endoscopic sinus surgery, catastrophic orbital bleeding and iatrogenic cerebrospinal fluid leak are the two serious complications surgeons most fear. This article discusses these avoidable complications and provides treatment algorithms for intraoperative maneuvers. A thorough understanding of the anatomy of the paranasal sinuses and their relationships with the anterior skull base, appropriate preoperative planning, and meticulous surgical technique are essential for preventing intraoperative cerebrospinal fluid leaks. Intraoperative orbital hematoma is discussed and a stepwise approach to reduce complications is provided.

Temporal bone fractures occur from high-energy mechanisms, typically but not limited to motor vehicle accidents. However, as the automotive industry continues to introduce improved safety measures, violence and falls account for a larger proportion of cases. Given the great forces involved, temporal bone fractures rarely occur in isolation and initial evaluation must focus on the fundamental ABCs of Advanced Trauma Life Support with special attention to Glasgow Coma Scale, intracranial injury, and cervical spine injury. Subsequent evaluation relies on physical examination, high-resolution CT, and electrodiagnostic testing to address the neurotologic consequences of temporal bone fracture, including cerebrospinal fluid leak, facial nerve injury, and injury to the peripheral hearing and balance organs. Management algorithms must address immediate (eg, ABCs, neurosurgical issues), short-term (eg, cerebrospinal fluid leak, facial nerve injury, hearing loss), long-term (eg, facial nerve injury, hearing loss, vestibular injury), and delayed (eg, encephalocele, cholesteatoma, late meningitis) issues. This article reviews the current state of temporal bone fracture evaluation and management with special attention to mechanisms of injury, clinical presentations and emergency evaluation, and diagnostic workup, including the evolution of radiographic fracture classification systems and electrodiagnostic testing. Discussion of treatment approaches address management of immediate, short-term, long-term, and delayed complications.

Emotions are communicated through facial expression. Happiness, confusion, and frustration can be expressed with a slight smile, eyebrow shift, or wrinkled nose. Injury to the facial nerve and subsequent inability of perform volitional mimetic movement can provoke anxiety. This article explores the causes, treatment, and prevention of facial nerve paralysis.

Sudden sensorineural hearing loss is a medical emergency in search of an appropriate treatment. Almost all aspects of this disease process are disputed in the literature. The natural course of the disease process has not been well defined, although spontaneous recovery in a percentage of patients appears well accepted. Little scientific data exist to develop an evidence-based treatment protocol. The more common elements of treatment in the United States include oral steroid therapy, transtympanic steroid therapy, and potentially oral antiviral therapy. Other therapies are used with great frequency, and their potential should not be discounted.

FORTHCOMING ISSUES

August 2008

Laryngeal Cancer
Nasir Bhatti, MD and Ralph Tufano, MD,
Guest Editors

October 2008

Pediatric Laryngeal Reconstruction
Peter Koltai, MD, *Guest Editor*

December 2008

Revision Thyroid Surgery
David Goldberg, MD, *Guest Editor*

RECENT ISSUES

April 2008

The Unified Airway
John H. Krouse, MD, PhD, *Guest Editor*

February 2008

Imaging of the Head and Neck
Barton Branstetter MD, *Guest Editor*

December 2007

**Life-Long Learning in Otolaryngology Practice:
From GME to MOC**
Matthew W. Ryan, MD and
Francis B. Quinn, Jr, MD, FACS, MS(ICS),
Guest Editors

The Clinics are now available online!

Access your subscription at
www.theclinics.com

Otolaryngol Clin N Am
41 (2008) xiii–xiv

Preface

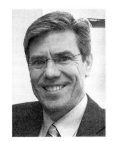 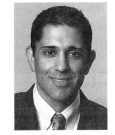

John L. Dornhoffer, MD   Rakesh K. Chandra, MD
Guest Editors

The head and neck is an anatomic crossroads of multiple functions critical to human well being, including respiration, digestion, sensation, communication, and aesthetics. Diseases that acutely threaten these vital systems can have catastrophic consequences, including impairment of interpersonal interaction, disfigurement, and loss of life. As with any emergency situation, attention must be devoted to the priorities of management: airway, breathing, circulation, and disability. Otolaryngic emergencies may manifest at each of these levels in the form of acute airway obstruction, epistaxis, and the gamut of traumatic, infectious, and inflammatory disorders that affect special sensation, neurologic function, and cosmesis. Therefore, the management of head and neck emergencies requires a diversity of skills and a broad knowledge base.

> It stands to the everlasting credit of science that by acting on the human mind it has overcome man's insecurity before himself and before nature.
> —Albert Einstein

In a field as diverse as otolaryngology, it is beyond the scope of this issue of *Otolaryngologic Clinics of North America,* and perhaps most text books, to provide a comprehensive treatise of all emergencies involving the ears, nose, and throat. We have attempted to bring in experts from our respective fields to describe those conditions that require urgent evaluation and treatment, but are also relatively common.

0030-6665/08/$ - see front matter © 2008 Elsevier Inc. All rights reserved.
doi:10.1016/j.otc.2008.01.010   *oto.theclinics.com*

Otolaryngology as a specialty continues to evolve with advances in science and technology. The keystone skill of the otolaryngologist has been the ability to see and work in dark or narrow areas, and the evolution of endoscopy, optics, and radiologic imaging has markedly augmented our capabilities. These modalities have permitted earlier diagnosis, detailed anatomic assessment, and minimally invasive surgery: philosophies that can be extended to the emergency setting. Unfortunately, there is very little overlap between our specialty and other branches of surgery or medicine regarding the intensive training required to manage the conditions reviewed in this issue. Stated another way, many of these entities remain the exclusive domain of the otolaryngologist, and the articles presented strive to keep practitioners at the forefront in the management of these disorders.

Where evidence-based medicine is lacking, such as in sudden sensorineural hearing loss and facial nerve injury, the authors have done an excellent job in presenting not only comprehensive reviews of the controversies, but also logical treatment algorithms based on their experience. It is hoped that this issue of *Otolaryngologic Clinics of North America*, entitled "ENT Emergencies," will be useful for the otolaryngologist as well as the general practitioner and emergency physician.

John L. Dornhoffer, MD
Division of Neurotology
Department of Otolaryngology/Head and Neck Surgery
University of Arkansas for Medical Sciences
4301 West Markham, Slot 543
Little Rock, AK 72205, USA

E-mail address: dornhofferjohnl@uams.edu

Rakesh K. Chandra, MD
Northwestern Sinus & Allergy Center
Department of Otolaryngology/Head and Neck Surgery
Northwestern University, Feinberg School of Medicine
303 East Chicago Avenue
Chicago, IL 60611-3008, USA

E-mail address: rickchandra@hotmail.edu

ELSEVIER
SAUNDERS

Otolaryngol Clin N Am
41 (2008) xv

OTOLARYNGOLOGIC
CLINICS
OF NORTH AMERICA

Dedication

from Rakesh K. Chandra, MD

I would like to dedicate this volume to my wife, Karyn, and my daughters, Kathryn and Sabrina. My family has been a steadfast source of inspiration, motivation, and support throughout my career.

doi:10.1016/j.otc.2008.01.011

imaging to confirm that no abscess cavity has been missed and obviate the need for dangerous surgical exploration. Abscesses that spread into adjacent deep neck spaces and those that involve the poststyloid compartment require an external cervical approach to incision and drainage.

Masticator/temporal space

The masticator space lies between the medial pterygoid muscle and the more lateral masseter muscle, and is enclosed by the divisions of the superficial layer of deep cervical fascia that envelop these muscles. It extends back to the posterior aspect of the mandible and superiorly as the temporal space, to surround the temporalis muscle deep to the temporalis fascia. Its contents include the temporalis muscle, the ramus of the mandible, divisions of the mandibular nerve (V_3), and the internal maxillary artery. Most masticator space infections originate from the posterior mandibular molars; less common sources include trauma and surgery. Patients often present with severe trismus, sore throat, dysphagia, pain surrounding the ramus of the mandible, and preauricular or mandibular swelling. More extensive infections can cause swelling of the entire side of the face, and involvement of the orbit may lead to proptosis, optic neuritis, and cranial nerve VI palsy. The surgical approach to incision and drainage of the masticator space depends on the location of the abscess in relation to the mandible. An intraoral approach at the retromolar trigone is appropriate for draining abscesses medial to the ramus of the mandible, and an extraoral approach along the inferior border of the mandible is used for draining abscesses lateral to the mandibular ramus. An incision through the temporalis fascia along the hairline is necessary to drain abscesses that spread superiorly and surround the temporalis muscle within the temporal space [1,4].

Buccal space

The buccal space lies between the buccopharyngeal fascia overlying the buccinator muscle medially and the skin of the cheek laterally, and is limited inferiorly by the border of the mandible and posteriorly by the pterygomandibular raphe. It contains the buccal fat pad, the parotid duct, and the facial artery. Most buccal space infections are odontogenic in origin and present with a warm and tender swelling within the cheek and minimal systemic symptoms. Trismus may be present if the infection spreads posteriorly to involve the masseter muscle [1,4].

Parotid space

The parotid space exists within the capsule that is formed by the superficial layer of deep cervical fascia as it envelops the parotid gland. The fascia on the medial aspect of the gland is thin and provides little resistance to the spread of parotid space infections into the adjacent parapharyngeal space. In addition to the parotid gland, the space also contains the facial nerve, external carotid artery, retromandibular vein, auriculotemporal nerve, superficial temporal artery, and lymph nodes. Parotid space infections often result from parotid duct obstruction or suppurative lymphadenitis, and occasionally originate from odontogenic infections of the mandibular molars that traverse the masticator space. Afflicted patients usually present with severe pain and swelling at the angle of the mandible, but little or no trismus unless the masticator space is sufficiently involved. Systemic symptoms such as fever and chills may accompany the spread of infection into the parapharyngeal space and other deep neck spaces. An external, parotidectomy-like approach is used to drain a parotid space abscess, and blunt dissection, either superior or inferior to the posterior belly of the digastric muscle, allows concurrent drainage of the parapharyngeal space when it is involved [1,4].

Spaces that involve the entire length of the neck

Retropharyngeal space

The retropharyngeal (retrovisceral, retroesophageal) space lies between the visceral (buccopharyngeal) fascia covering the posterior pharynx and esophagus and the alar fascia, a division of the deep layer of deep cervical fascia, and occupies the space posterior to the pharynx and esophagus. It extends from the base of the skull down into the mediastinum, where the visceral and alar fascias fuse at the level of the second thoracic vertebra. Laterally, it is bounded by the carotid sheaths. The retropharyngeal space is fused down the midline and contains two chains of lymph nodes extending down each side. Retropharyngeal abscesses are unilateral as a result of the midline fusion, and are primarily seen early in childhood because these lymph nodes tend to regress with age. Upper respiratory infections cause most retropharyngeal disease in children because these lymph nodes receive drainage from the nose, sinuses, and pharynx. Retropharyngeal infection is also seen in children and adults following trauma to the posterior pharynx or as an extension from an adjacent parapharyngeal space infection [4]. Cultures of retropharyngeal aspirates are generally polymicrobial and contain common oropharyngeal flora such as *S viridans* [16], with the exception that young children are more likely to be infected with pathogenic *Streptococcus* species and *Staphylococcus aureus* [5].

Children with retropharyngeal infections often present with neck pain, neck swelling, fever, irritability, dysphagia, excessive drooling, and dyspnea or noisy breathing suggestive of upper airway compromise [4,16]. Adults tend to present with neck pain, fever, anorexia, nasal obstruction, snoring, and dyspnea [1]. Careful oropharyngeal examination often reveals unilateral bulging of the posterior pharynx, which is localized in retropharyngeal lymphadenitis and may extend the length of the pharynx when cellulitis or an abscess is present. In the absence of acute distress, CECT of the head and neck can be used to confirm the diagnosis and evaluate for spread of infection into adjacent deep neck spaces [4].

The most feared complications of retropharyngeal infection are airway obstruction and rupture of an abscess with subsequent aspiration of pus. Patients who have signs of airway compromise should be taken immediately to the operating room before being examined. With the patient in the head-down Trendelenburg's position and intubated along the opposite side of the pharynx from the swelling, needle aspiration should precede intraoral incision and drainage, to obtain specimens for culture and sensitivity and to minimize any risk of the patient aspirating pus during the procedure. Spread of the infection into the parapharyngeal space may necessitate an external cervical approach to incision and drainage if the involvement is not confined to the prestyloid compartment medial to the great vessels [4].

Danger space

The danger space lies posterior to the retropharyngeal space between the alar and prevertebral fascias, the two divisions of the deep layer of deep cervical fascia, and extends from the skull base down into the posterior mediastinum to the level of the diaphragm. Infections here indirectly result from the spread of retropharyngeal, parapharyngeal, and prevertebral space abscesses. The "danger" lies in the tendency for infections to spread inferiorly through the space and into the thorax because the loose areolar contents offer little resistance, resulting in complications such as mediastinitis, empyema, and sepsis. Danger space infections initially present in the same way as retropharyngeal infections, and CECT is necessary to differentiate between them [1].

Prevertebral space

The prevertebral space is a potential space between the prevertebral fascia and the underlying vertebral bodies and deep cervical musculature. It extends down the entire length of the vertebral column to the coccyx. However, dense fibrous attachments between the prevertebral fascia and deep cervical muscles tend to contain prevertebral infections and help prevent longitudinal spread. Sources of infection include trauma to the posterior pharynx, and secondary spread from Pott's abscesses and retropharyngeal and danger space infections. Patients often present with a midline bulge in the posterior pharynx, in contrast to the unilateral bulge often seen in retropharyngeal infections. Complications include osteomyelitis and spinal instability, which require a prolonged course of antibiotics. Once identified with CECT, prevertebral space abscesses should be drained using an external cervical approach rather than an intraoral approach, which can lead to a persistent draining fistula in the posterior pharynx [4].

Carotid space

The carotid (visceral vascular) space lies within the carotid sheath and houses the carotid artery, internal jugular vein, cervical sympathetic chain, and cranial nerves IX, X, XI, and XII. It is similar to the prevertebral space in that it contains little areolar tissue, and thus is somewhat resistant to the longitudinal spread of infection. However, as the well-known expression "Lincoln's highway" suggests, the carotid sheath receives contributions from all three layers of deep cervical fascia, extends from the base of the skull into the mediastinum, and can potentially serve as a "highway" for infectious spread originating in any deep neck space. In addition to secondary spread from adjacent deep neck spaces, direct inoculation into the neck in intravenous drug abusers and iatrogenic causes such as central venous catheterization can lead to carotid space infections. Patients often present with stiffness and ipsilateral swelling of the neck, fever, chills, ipsilateral Horner's syndrome, vocal cord paralysis, and other complication-related findings. IJVT can cause intermittent spiking fevers, and carotid artery rupture may be preceded by sentinel bleeds from the ear, nose, or mouth. An external cervical approach is used for incision and drainage of the carotid space [1,4].

Space below the level of the hyoid

Anterior visceral space

The anterior visceral (pretracheal) space is the only deep neck space limited to below the hyoid bone. It is bounded by the visceral division of the middle layer of deep cervical fascia and lies between the infrahyoid strap muscles and the esophagus. It contains the thyroid gland, the trachea, and the anterior wall of the esophagus, and extends from the thyroid cartilage down into the superior mediastinum overlying the aortic arch and fibrous pericardium. The anterior visceral and retropharyngeal spaces are separated by lateral attachments of the esophagus to the prevertebral fascia beginning at the level of the thyroid gland, so that the anterior visceral space lies anterior and the retropharyngeal space lies posterior to the esophagus [4].

Infections of the anterior visceral space often originate from traumatic perforation of the anterior esophageal wall and, less commonly, from neck trauma or thyroiditis. They often present with neck swelling, sore throat, dysphagia, hoarseness, and dyspnea as a result of pharyngeal, laryngeal, and supraglottic edema, which can potentially progress to airway compromise. In addition, the perforation of visceral contents may cause crepitation of the anterior neck, mediastinitis, and pneumothorax [4]. Boscolo-Rizzo and colleagues [17] noted that every infection involving the anterior visceral space in their study developed life-threatening complications, including five out of the six cases of mediastinitis that were encountered. Abscesses in the anterior visceral space require an external cervical approach to incision and drainage [4].

Diagnosing deep neck infection

History, physical examination, laboratory work, and diagnostic imaging each provide important clues when assessing a patient for DNI. However, initial evaluation of the airway is the first priority and any signs of respiratory distress or impending airway compromise should be immediately and aggressively managed. In the absence of a respiratory emergency, careful questioning should attempt to uncover potential sources of the infection, such as any recent illness, dental caries or procedures, trauma to the head and neck, or intravenous drug use. Risk factors, including diabetes mellitus, HIV infection, steroid therapy, chemotherapy, and other sources of immune dysfunction, should be identified early and appropriately managed to minimize potential complications.

Most studies of DNIs in the last decade recognized pain and swelling of the neck to be the most prevalent symptoms [6,17–21]. In other studies, odynophagia [22] and fever [23] were more frequently observed. Other common symptoms were space specific and included dysphagia, trismus, dysphonia, otalgia, and dyspnea. In the pediatric population, fever, neck mass, and neck stiffness were most prevalent, followed by sore throat, poor oral intake, drooling, and lymphadenopathy [16,24,25]. Infants less than 9 months old most often present with a neck mass or swelling, lymphadenopathy, fever, rhinorrhea, poor oral intake, and cough [26].

Initial laboratory work should include a complete blood count with differential, serum glucose, and electrolytes; coagulation studies (prothrombin time, partial thromboplastin time); HIV screening in adults; blood cultures; and appropriate cultures of aspirates obtained before antibiotics are instituted, if possible. Culture results are most accurate when obtained with needle aspiration, and specimens for anaerobic cultures should be placed immediately into an oxygen-free container. In addition to aerobic and anaerobic cultures, fungal and acid-fast cultures are recommended for immunocompromised patients [4]. Negative cultures, despite the finding of organisms on gram stain, may suggest an anaerobic infection [23]. Additional testing for atypical causes of DNI, such as *Bartonella henselae* (cat scratch disease), mycobacteria, or fungal infections, may be appropriate when cultures are negative [27].

Leukocytosis may correlate with the development of a drainable abscess, according to Miller and colleagues [12]. Leukopenia and persistent white blood cell counts of less than 8000 per mm^3 were noted by Har-El and colleagues [2] in most of their deep neck abscess patients who had concurrent HIV or tuberculosis infections.

Diagnostic imaging

Appropriate management of DNI is highly dependent on the location and extent of deep neck involvement, and diagnostic imaging is essential in nearly every case.

CECT has made an important contribution to characterizing the nature of a deep neck lesion, identifying the spaces involved, and aiding in the early recognition of complications. It is especially important in planning the surgical approach and is the current standard of care when managing

a suspected DNI [17]. In addition, CECT has been shown to identify imped-
ing airway complications before they present clinically [12,26]. Neck swelling that extends to the suprasternal notch may indicate involvement of
the mediastinum, and CECT should include the chest in such cases [19].
Serial CT scanning may be useful in monitoring patients who have mediastinitis [28]. When combined with careful clinical examination, CECT has
a reported accuracy of 89% in differentiating a drainable abscess from cellulitis [12]. CECT alone has an accuracy ranging from 63% [25] to 95% [14]
in making this distinction. Miller and colleagues [12] suggested that a discrete
hypodensity greater than 2 mL in volume on CECT is more predictive of
a deep neck abscess than the presence of a ring-enhancing lesion.

Plain films may also be of some use in certain cases of DNI. Chest radiograph is useful when screening for complications such as mediastinitis, pneumonia, and pleural effusion [19]. However, CECT is superior for evaluating
cellulitis or abscess within the mediastinum [6]. Lateral neck radiographs
have been used to screen for retropharyngeal and parapharyngeal abscesses.
Nagy and Backstrom [29] found them to have an 83% sensitivity, in comparison to 100% sensitivity for CECT, and recommended against the use
of lateral neck plain films in the workup of children with suspected DNIs.
Dental radiographs, such as the Panorex oral view, are useful in identifying
odontogenic sources of infection [1].

Ultrasound is more accurate than CECT in differentiating a drainable abscess from cellulitis [4]. In addition, it is portable, inexpensive, promptly
available at most institutions, and avoids exposure to radiation. However,
ultrasound is difficult to interpret, is subject to the skill level of the operator,
may not visualize deeper lesions, and does not provide the anatomic information necessary for planning the surgical approach to a DNI [30]. Therefore, ultrasound should be used to supplement CECT or MRI in cases when
the presence of a deep neck abscess is uncertain and to guide diagnostic and
therapeutic needle or catheter aspiration of superficial, uniloculated fluid
collections when imminent airway compromise is not evident [4].

MRI provides better soft tissue definition than CECT. In addition, MRI
avoids exposure to radiation, interference from dental fillings, and more al-
lergenic CT contrast material [1]. Magnetic resonance angiography (MRA)
it is especially useful in evaluating vascular complications, such as IJVT and
carotid artery aneurysm or rupture [23]. Unfortunately, the disadvantages of
MRI preclude its usefulness in most cases. MRI is expensive and requires
a lengthy scan time in comparison with CECT, which may necessitate sedation of a child or a distressed patient and increase the likelihood of airway
compromise [30].

Airway management

Acute airway obstruction is one of the most frequent and deadly complications of DNI. It is most often encountered in cases with multiple space

involvement, Ludwig's angina, or retropharyngeal, parapharyngeal, or anterior visceral space abscesses [18,31]. Studies by Har-El [2] and Parhiscar [32] found that up to 75% of cases of Ludwig's angina required a surgical airway, and the investigators recommended universal elective awake tracheostomy as a preventative measure in these patients. Tracheotomy under local anesthesia has been shown to be safe and effective [33], and is considered by some to be the standard of care for managing airway compromise in DNI patients [34]. Other methods of airway management include endotracheal intubation, fiber optic nasotracheal intubation, and cricothyrotomy. Each has advantages and disadvantages that must be carefully considered when selecting the safest and most appropriate method.

Careful monitoring of the airway is the first priority when treating any patient who has a DNI, and should continue for at least 48 hours after surgical intervention because of the potential for increased swelling in the postoperative period [23]. Indications for aggressive airway management include signs of respiratory distress (dyspnea, stridor, retractions) or impending airway compromise as noted on physical examination or diagnostic imaging (severe swelling within the pharynx, upward displacement of the tongue, airway edema, or airway compression by an abscess). In advanced cases of DNI, placing the patient in the supine position may precipitate complete airway obstruction, which is important to consider when sedating a supine patient or sending them for an MRI without first securing his or her airway [34]. Some investigators speculate that routine use of intravenous steroids in patients who have impending airway obstruction can minimize swelling and reduce the need for aggressive airway intervention [3,21,34]. However, systemic steroids have hyperglycemic effects and should be avoided in patients who have diabetes mellitus or poor glucose control.

Endotracheal intubation may be attempted before tracheotomy in most patients who have DNI. However, it is often made difficult by distorted airway anatomy, immobility of the soft tissues, or trismus that limits access to the mouth. Extreme care should be taken in the presence of a pharyngeal wall abscess because of the risk of rupture and subsequent aspiration of pus. In less severe infections, trismus may be overcome with the use of general anesthesia. However, in more advanced cases, general anesthesia is dangerous and can precipitate complete airway obstruction that necessitates an emergency tracheotomy [34]. The advantages of endotracheal intubation are fast airway control and avoidance of the risks associated with a surgical procedure. The disadvantages include difficulty in the presence of airway edema, patient discomfort, a less secure airway, greater need for patient sedation and mechanical ventilation, and potential for laryngotracheal stenosis. Unplanned extubation is the most common complication of endotracheal intubation. Both planned and unplanned extubation risk airway loss secondary to worsening laryngeal edema and subsequent inability to reintubate, which is an avoidable source of mortality. In comparison with patients who received tracheotomies, intubated patients have been shown to have longer hospital stays, spend more time in the ICU, have higher mortality from airway loss, and have 60% greater overall hospital expenses [35].

Fiber optic nasotracheal intubation, when performed by experienced hands using topical anesthesia, is especially useful in patients who have severe trismus but whose airways are otherwise uncompromised [23,34]. Fiber optic nasotracheal intubation is often made difficult by edema, copious secretions, inadequate experience, or improper application of topical anesthetic. However, in a study by Ovassapian and colleagues [34], all 25 attempts at fiber optic nasotracheal intubation in adult patients who had DNI were successful using careful titration of intravenous diazepam or midazolam with or without fentanyl to reduce laryngeal spasm before the application of topical anesthesia, which can have an irritating effect on the airway.

Tracheotomy under local anesthesia is indicated for severe or impending airway obstruction when trismus or massive soft tissue edema precludes endotracheal intubation or when repeated attempts at intubation have failed [4,33]. Separate incisions should be used for tracheotomy and drainage procedures of the anterior neck to avoid infectious spread into the mediastinum [6]. Tracheotomy should be avoided if possible when the pretracheal or anterior visceral space is involved in the infection [23]. The advantages of tracheotomy include airway security, less need for sedation, and earlier transfer to a noncritical care unit. In addition, tracheotomy patients have been shown to have shorter hospital stays, spend less time in the ICU, have 60% less overall hospital expenses, and have lower mortality due to loss of the airway, when compared with patients who underwent endotracheal intubation. The disadvantages of tracheotomy include surgical risks such as bleeding and pneumothorax, and the potential of causing tracheal stenosis [35]. Other reported risks of tracheotomy in DNI patients include mediastinitis, aspiration of pus, airway loss, rupture of the innominate artery, and death [34].

Cricothyrotomy, or emergency tracheotomy, can provide urgent airway access when complete loss of the airway necessitates immediate surgical intervention. The rigid nature of the thyroid and cricoid cartilages limits the size of the tube that can be placed to an average of 9.0 mm in diameter. Passage of the cricothyrotomy tube may cause trauma to the posterior wall of the trachea, and subglottic stenosis is a potential complication. Cricothyrotomy should be converted to a standard tracheotomy within 24 to 48 hours [33].

Microbiology

Cultures of aspirates from deep neck abscesses are commonly polymicrobial and reflect the oropharyngeal flora and odontogenic nature of these infections. Frequently isolated aerobes include *S viridans*, *Klebsiella pneumoniae*, and *S aureus*, and, less frequently, *Streptococcus pneumoniae*, *Streptococcus pyogenes*, *Neisseria* species, and *Haemophilus influenzae*. Common anaerobic isolates include *Peptostreptococcus*, *Bacteroides fragilis*, pigmented *Prevotella* and *Porphyromonas* spp, *Fusobacterium* spp, and *Eikenella corrodens* (see Refs. [1,2,24,32,36,37]). Anaerobic bacteria are increasingly penicillin resistant because of production of β-lactamase, which is released into the infection and has a protective effect for nearby penicillin-sensitive species [36]. *E corrodens*, an anaerobe frequently isolated in children and intravenous drug abusers, is universally resistant to clindamycin and metronidazole, but is sensitive to penicillin and aminoglycosides [24,38]. In addition, methicillin-resistant *S aureus* (MRSA), once considered a nosocomial infection, has been seen with increasing prevalence as a community-acquired cause of DNI in intravenous drug abusers, immunocompromised patients, infants, and young children (see Refs. [16,24,26,28,38,39]), and in certain geographic areas MRSA is an emerging pathogen in necrotizing fasciitis and descending mediastinitis [28,40]. *K pneumoniae* is consistently the most common cause of DNI in patients who have poorly controlled diabetes mellitus [20,21,31].

Empiric antibiotic coverage

Every patient who has a DNI should be given initial empiric antibiotic therapy until culture and sensitivity results are available. Empiric therapy should be effective against the aerobic and anaerobic bacteria that are commonly involved, and, once available, the results of the culture and sensitivity tests can allow for tailoring of adequate antibiotic therapy. Either penicillin in combination with a β-lactamase inhibitor (such as amoxicillin or ticarcillin with clavulanic acid) or a β-lactamase–resistant antibiotic (such as cefoxitin, cefuroxime, imipenem, or meropenem) in combination with a drug that is highly effective against most anaerobes (such as clindamycin or metronidazole) is recommended for optimal empiric coverage [6,17,21,36]. Vancomycin should be considered for empiric therapy in intravenous drug abusers at risk for infection with MRSA [1,38] and in patients who have profound neutropenia or immune dysfunction [39]. Ceftriaxone and clindamycin can be used as empiric therapy against community-acquired MRSA in young children to ensure adequate coverage and avoid resistance to vancomycin [28]. The addition of gentamicin for effective gram-negative coverage against *K pneumoniae*, which is resistant to clindamycin, is highly recommended for diabetic patients [21,41]; however, renal function should be closely monitored whenever aminoglycosides are administered to patients at risk for renal disease. Parenteral antibiotic therapy should be continued until the patient has been afebrile for at least 48 hours, followed by oral therapy using amoxicillin with clavulanic acid, clindamycin, ciprofloxacin, trimethoprim-sulfamethoxazole, or metronidazole [1,36].

Conservative medical management

Surgical drainage is the classic approach to any DNI with suspected abscess formation and is still felt by many investigators to be the first-line treatment in such cases [23,27,32]. Recent studies, however, are beginning to show that, in select cases, an uncomplicated deep neck abscess or cellulitis can be effectively treated with antibiotics and careful monitoring, without surgical drainage. Simultaneous medical treatment for associated comorbidities such as diabetes can improve the overall immune status of a DNI patient. A study by Mayor and colleagues [22] found that conservative treatment does not increase mortality or length of hospitalization in DNI. The use of steroids along with antibiotic treatment may reduce the need for surgical intervention by minimizing airway edema, inflammation, and the progression of cellulitis into an abscess [21,22]. A study by Oh and associates [11] found that 55.9% of 34 parapharyngeal space abscesses responded well to conservative medical management. Thompson and colleagues [37] noted that 25% of children with retropharyngeal abscesses responded to medical treatment and did not require surgical drainage. However, conservative management may not be appropriate for diabetic patients who have demonstrated a lack of response to such treatment [17]. Aspiration of an abscess for culture and sensitivity is recommended for immunocompromised patients and anyone at risk for infection with an unusual or atypical pathogen [4].

Surgical intervention

Surgical intervention remains the mainstay of treatment for more complicated or severe cases of DNI. Indications for surgery include airway compromise, critical condition, septicemia, complications, descending infection, diabetes mellitus, or no clinical improvement within 48 hours of the initiation of parenteral antibiotics [1,4,17,31]. In addition, abscesses greater than 3 cm in diameter that involve the prevertebral, anterior visceral, or carotid spaces, or that involve more than two spaces, should be surgically drained [17]. Surgical drainage can be performed in several ways, including simple intraoral or extraoral incision and drainage for superficial abscesses, a more extensive external cervical approach for deeper and more complicated infections, and minimally invasive techniques such as image-guided needle aspiration and indwelling catheter placement. Abscesses that are small and unilocular may respond well to needle aspiration, whereas larger and multilocular abscesses usually require incision and drainage [4]. Regardless of the approach, a surgical specimen (either aspirated pus or debrided tissue) should be obtained and sent for gram stain and cultures as soon as the abscess cavity is entered. Swabs are generally avoided because they prevent accurate culturing of anaerobic bacteria from the wound. Fluid resuscitation before surgery is important in DNI patients because these patients frequently present in a dehydrated state [1].

The external cervical approach is most often used when draining the anterior visceral, submandibular, parapharyngeal, prevertebral, and carotid spaces, and for complicated retropharyngeal abscesses that cannot be fully drained using an intraoral approach [4]. Wide exposure of the infected tissue is important, as is debridement of any necrotic tissue that is present. Wounds requiring extensive debridement should be left open and packed with antimicrobial dressings to allow for frequent inspection. Wounds with less necrosis can be closed at surgery with active suction drainage. In cases involving descending infections, cervical drainage is sufficient as long as the infection remains above the carina. Transthoracic drainage is necessary when infection spreads below the carina [1].

Minimally invasive techniques have been used more recently for well-defined, unilocular abscesses in patients who do not have airway compromise. Ultrasound guidance is appropriate for locating and draining abscesses accessible through the skin, and CT guidance is helpful when attempting needle aspiration of a deep, difficult to access collection of fluid. Needle aspiration and catheter placement offer the advantages of a small point of entry, quick healing time, little or no scar formation, and less risk of contaminating the surrounding deep neck spaces while draining pus. A study by Yeow and colleagues [42] arbitrarily used ultrasound-guided needle aspiration for unilocular abscesses measuring less than 3 cm in diameter, and ultrasound-guided catheter placement for unilocular abscesses measuring greater than 3 cm in diameter, extending into deep neck spaces, or located within a glandular structure. Needle aspiration was repeated within 3 days when residual purulent discharge was observed. Catheters with continuous suction were left in place for 3 to 5 days. Successful percutaneous treatment was defined by the disappearance of the abscess, as documented by follow-up ultrasound, CECT, or clinical improvement. Failure of percutaneous treatment was recognized and subsequently converted to open drainage when the abscess remained unchanged or increased in size, when signs of systemic toxicity persisted, or after two attempts at needle aspiration failed. Of 15 patients with deep neck abscesses, 8 of 10 were successfully treated with ultrasound-guided needle aspiration and 5 of 5 were successfully treated using ultrasound-guided catheter placement, for an overall success rate of 87% using minimally invasive techniques.

Complications

Mediastinitis results from downward extension of an infection that involves the spaces that extend the length of the neck or the anterior visceral space [23]. The causative organism varies, depending on the origin of the infection; most cases are polymicrobial and involve both aerobes and anaerobes [20]. A recent study by Naidu and colleagues [28] found MRSA to be the cause of descending mediastinitis in a 4-month-old child, which resulted in significant respiratory distress and hemodynamic instability but responded eventually to surgical drainage, vancomycin, and rifampin therapy. Afflicted patients will frequently complain of increasing chest pain or dyspnea, and chest radiography or CECT may demonstrate a widened mediastinum or pneumomediastinum [23]. Transthoracic drainage is necessary when the infection spreads below the carina [1]. In one study, the mortality rate for patients who had mediastinitis was 40% [31].

Lemierre syndrome, or suppurative thrombophlebitis of the internal jugular vein, results from extension of the infection into the carotid space. Pathognomonic findings include swelling and tenderness at the angle of the jaw and along the SCM muscle, along with signs of sepsis (spiking fevers, chills) and evidence of pulmonary emboli [43]. IJVT may be detected using high-resolution ultrasound, CECT, or MRI/MRA. Treatment involves prolonged antimicrobial therapy directed by culture and sensitivity results, and anticoagulation is currently recommended for 3 months when thrombus progression or septic emboli are present. Most cases resolve with antibiotic and anticoagulation therapy and do not require surgical ligation and resection of the internal jugular vein [43,44]. Fibrinolytic agents may be used if IJVT is recognized within 4 days of onset, but they carry a higher risk of hemorrhage than anticoagulation. Endovascular stenting is another option for patients able to tolerate long-term anticoagulation, and superior vena cava filters have reportedly been used in select cases [44].

Carotid artery aneurysm or rupture may present with a pulsatile neck mass and often results in four cardinal signs:

• Recurrent sentinel hemorrhages from the pharynx or ear
• Protracted clinical course (7–14 days)
• Hematoma of the surrounding neck tissues
• Hemodynamic collapse

Early recognition and surgical intervention to gain proximal control of the common carotid artery is essential because more distal ligation may be impossible [23]. Interventional radiologic procedures such as endovascular stenting or vessel occlusion are also an option in less urgent cases.

Necrotizing cervical fasciitis is a fulminant infection that spreads along fascial planes and causes necrosis of connective tissues (Fig. 4). The pathogens involved are usually polymicrobial and odontogenic, and they include *S pyogenes*, *Clostridium perfringens*, and mixed aerobes and anaerobes. MRSA has recently been recognized as an important cause and may necessitate the addition of vancomycin to empiric treatment of this condition [1,40]. Patients who have necrotizing fasciitis are acutely ill with high fevers, and the skin overlying the necrosis may be tender, edematous, and erythematous, with indistinct transition to normal skin. Soft tissue crepitation due to infection with gas-producing organisms may be present, and, in more advanced cases, the skin becomes pale, anesthetic, and dusky, with blistering and sloughing [1]. CECT may demonstrate diffuse cellulitis with infiltration of the skin and subcutaneous tissues, and myositis, compartmental fluid,

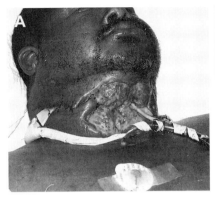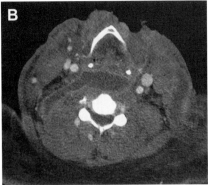

Fig. 4. Diabetic patient with severe, complicated DNI involving multiple spaces. (*A*) The swelling and necrosis often seen with cervical necrotizing fasciitis. (*B*) CT scan of the same patient, showing widespread extension of a deep neck abscess.

and gas accumulations [45]. Managing necrotizing fasciitis is best accomplished in an ICU and involves parenteral antibiotics along with early and frequent surgical debridement of any devitalized tissue. The wound should be left open and packed with antimicrobial dressings until the infection has subsided. Hyperbaric oxygen is useful as an adjunctive treatment in hemodynamically stable patients. The condition is often accompanied by mediastinitis and sepsis, which increase the risk of mortality [1].

Aspiration pneumonia, lung abscess, empyema, and even asphyxiation may result when an abscess ruptures into the larynx or trachea and purulent drainage is subsequently aspirated. Horner's syndrome and cranial nerve IX through XII palsies result from infections that invade the carotid space. Osteomyelitis can involve the mandible or cervical vertebral bodies, and can lead to vertebral subluxation [4]. Sepsis is often cited as a direct cause of mortality in DNI studies [19,27,31,46]. Other potential complications include meningitis, intracranial abscess, and disseminated intravascular coagulation.

Risk factors

Diabetes mellitus is frequently cited as the most common associated systemic disease in DNI studies (see Refs. [17,20,21,27,31,32]). Hyperglycemia has been found to impair neutrophil function [47,48] and the complement pathway, and increase the virulence of certain pathogens [48]. The immune dysfunction resulting from uncontrolled diabetes diminishes the ability to confine an infection, which is evident in the frequency of multispace involvement in diabetics with DNIs [17,49,50]. *K pneumoniae* is the most frequently isolated pathogen from deep neck aspirates in diabetic patients (see Refs. [20,21,31,49,50]), and is effectively treated by adding gentamicin to their empiric antibiotic therapy [21]. Diabetics tend to develop DNIs at an older age [49,50], have lengthier hospitalizations [17,20,21,49,50], require more frequent surgical intervention [49], respond poorly to conservative medical therapy [17,50], and develop complications with greater frequency, when compared with nondiabetic patients (see Fig. 4) [17,49,50]. Therefore, management of DNI in diabetic patients should include earlier and more aggressive medical and surgical therapies and careful monitoring to maintain blood glucose levels below 200 mg/dL [31,50].

Immunosuppression from other sources such as HIV infection, chemotherapy, chronic renal failure, hepatic disease, and chronic steroid therapy for autoimmune disease also places a patient at increased risk for more severe and atypical infections of the head and neck. Immunocompromised patients are more likely to present with minimal signs and symptoms despite a greater risk for complications. DNI may be the first clinical manifestation of an HIV infection, and the laboratory work for unknown at-risk patients should include an HIV screening panel. AIDS patients who have more advanced immune dysfunction often have low or normal white blood cell counts regardless of the severity of their infections [32]. Empiric antibiotic therapy should be expanded to cover for all potential pathogens the immunocompromised patient is at risk for, and every effort should be made to identify the infectious agents to direct proper treatment [1].

Intravenous drug abuse places a patient at risk for carotid space infection when the neck is used as an injection site. Pathogens are introduced through the skin, and an abscess may form around a foreign body such as a broken needle [1]. Although the overall incidence of intravenous drug abuse may be declining in some areas [32], these patients have a much higher infection rate with resistant organisms such as MRSA and *E corrodens*. Therefore, appropriate empiric antibiotic coverage should include vancomycin along with adequate anaerobic coverage that is also effective against *E corrodens*, such as ciprofloxacin or an aminoglycoside [1,38].

Congenital cysts should be suspected in any patient who has recurrence of a DNI. Congenital lesions include branchial cleft cysts, lymphangiomas, thyroglossal duct cysts, and cervical thymic cysts. Infection in any of these cysts may present similarly with a painful, tender swelling in the neck and variable degrees of overlying cellulitis. CECT is useful in early recognition and surgical planning, but definitive diagnosis requires surgical confirmation. Initially, infections within congenital cysts may respond well to antibiotic therapy. However, complete surgical excision of the cyst wall is absolutely necessary to prevent the inevitable recurrence of infection [51].

Primary head and neck malignancy presented initially as DNI in several recent cases. These patients were generally older, ranging in age from 40 to 74 years. They presented similarly to any other patient with DNI, except that, with careful questioning, most were found to have clinical symptoms related to their tumors such as pre-existing small neck masses [52]. In another scenario, repeat biopsies in patients who had refractory lymphadenopathy despite adequate DNI treatment eventually revealed malignancies [21]. Therefore, it has been recommended that the workup of adult patients who have risk factors for primary head and neck malignancy include a careful history, a comprehensive ear, nose, and throat examination, including panendoscopy, and pathologic examination of tissue obtained surgically or by needle aspiration [27,52].

References

[1] Weed HG, Forest LA. Deep neck infection. In: Cummings CW, Flint PW, Harker LA, et al, editors. Otolaryngology: head and neck surgery, vol. 3. 4th edition. Philadelphia: Elsevier Mosby; 2005. p. 2515–24.

[2] Har-El G, Aroesty J, Shaha A, et al. Changing trends in deep neck abscess: a retrospective study of 110 patients. Oral Surg Oral Med Oral Pathol 1994;77(5):446–50.

[3] Larawin V, Naipao J, Dubey S. Head and neck space infections. Otolaryngol Head Neck Surg 2006;135(6):889–93.

[4] Yellon RF. Head and neck space infections. In: Bluestone CD, Casselbrant ML, Stool SE, et al, editors. Pediatric otolaryngology, vol. 2. 4th edition. Philadelphia: Saunders; 2003. p. 1681–701.

[5] Brook I. Microbiology and management of peritonsillar, retropharyngeal, and parapharyngeal abscesses. J Oral Maxillofac Surg 2004;62:1545–50.

[6] Stalfors J, Adielsson A, Ebenfelt A, et al. Deep neck space infections remain a surgical challenge: a study of 72 patients. Acta Otolaryngol 2004;124(10):1191–6.

[7] Rega A, Aziz S, Ziccardi V. Microbiology and antibiotic sensitivities of head and neck space infections of odontogenic origin. J Oral Maxillofac Surg 2006;64(9):1377–80.

[8] Wasson J, Hopkins C, Bowdler D. Did Ludwig's angina kill Ludwig? J Laryngol Otol 2006; 120(5):363–5.

[9] Bross-Soriano D, Arrieta-Gomez J, Prado-Calleros H, et al. Management of Ludwig's angina with small neck incisions: 18 years experience. Otolaryngol Head Neck Surg 2004; 130(6):712–7.

[10] Shockley W. Ludwig angina: a review of current airway management. Arch Otolaryngol Head Neck Surg 1999;125(5):596–9.

[11] Oh J, Kim Y, Kim C. Parapharyngeal abscess: comprehensive management protocol. ORL J Otorhinolaryngol Relat Spec 2007;69(1):37–42.

[12] Miller W, Furst I, Sandor G, et al. A prospective, blinded comparison of clinical examination and computed tomography in deep neck infections. Laryngoscope 1999;109(11):1873–9.

[13] Sichel J, Attal P, Hocwald E, et al. Redefining parapharyngeal space infections. Ann Otol Rhinol Laryngol 2006;115(2):117–23.

[14] Nagy M, Pizzuto M, Backstrom J, et al. Deep neck infections in children: a new approach to diagnosis and treatment. Laryngoscope 1997;107(12):1627–34.

[15] Cable B, Brenner P, Bauman N, et al. Image-guided surgical drainage of medial parapharyngeal abscesses in children: a novel adjuvant to a difficult approach. Ann Otol Rhinol Laryngol 2004;113(2):115–20.

[16] Tan P, Chang L, Huang Y, et al. Deep neck infections in children. J Microbiol Immunol Infect 2001;34(4):287–92.

[17] Boscolo-Rizzo P, Marchiori C, Zanetti F, et al. Conservative management of deep neck abscesses in adults: the importance of CECT findings. Otolaryngol Head Neck Surg 2006; 135(6):894–9.

[18] Boscolo-Rizzo P, Marchiori C, Montolli F, et al. Deep neck infections: a constant challenge. ORL J Otorhinolaryngol Relat Spec 2006;68(5):259–65.

[19] Crespo A, Chone C, Fonseca A, et al. Clinical versus computed tomography evaluation in the diagnosis and management of deep neck infection. Sao Paulo Med J 2004;122(6): 259–63.

[20] Lee J, Kim H, Lim S. Predisposing factors of complicated deep neck infection: an analysis of 158 cases. Yonsei Med J 2007;48(1):55–62.

[21] Wang L, Kuo W, Tsai S, et al. Characterizations of life-threatening deep cervical space infections: a review of one hundred ninety-six cases. Am J Otolaryngol 2003;24(2):111–7.

[22] Mayor G, Millan J, Martinez-Vidal A. Is conservative treatment of deep neck space infections appropriate? Head Neck 2001;23(2):126–33.

[23] Gidley P, Ghorayeb B, Stiernberg C. Contemporary management of deep neck space infections. Otolaryngol Head Neck Surg 1997;116(1):16–22.

[24] Coticchia J, Getnick G, Yun R, et al. Age-, site-, and time-specific differences in pediatric deep neck abscesses. Arch Otolaryngol Head Neck Surg 2004;130(2):201–7.

[25] Vural C, Gungor A, Comerci S. Accuracy of computerized tomography in deep neck infections in the pediatric population. Am J Otolaryngol 2003;24(3):143–8.

[26] Cmejrek R, Coticchia J, Arnold J. Presentation, diagnosis, and management of deep-neck abscesses in infants. Arch Otolaryngol Head Neck Surg 2002;128(12):1361–4.

[27] Ridder G, Technau-Ihling K, Sander A, et al. Spectrum and management of deep neck space infections: an 8-year experience of 234 cases. Otolaryngol Head Neck Surg 2005;133(5): 709–14.

[28] Naidu S, Donepudi S, Stocks R, et al. Methicillin-resistant Staphylococcus aureus as a pathogen in deep neck abscesses: a pediatric case series. Int J Pediatr Otorhinolaryngol 2005; 69(10):1367–71.

[29] Nagy M, Backstrom J. Comparison of the sensitivity of lateral neck radiographs and computed tomography scanning in pediatric deep-neck infections. Laryngoscope 1999;109(5): 775–9.

[30] Smith J, Hsu J, Chang J. Predicting deep neck space abscess using computed tomography. Am J Otolaryngol 2006;27(4):244–7.

[31] Huang T, Liu T, Chen P, et al. Deep neck infection: analysis of 185 cases. Head Neck 2004; 26(10):854–60.

[32] Parhiscar A, Har-El G. Deep neck abscess: a retrospective review of 210 cases. Ann Otol Rhinol Laryngol 2001;110(11):1051–4.

[33] Yuen H, Loy A, Johari S. Urgent awake tracheotomy for impending airway obstruction. Otolaryngol Head Neck Surg 2007;136(5):838–42.

[34] Ovassapian A, Tuncbilek M, Weitzel E, et al. Airway management in adult patients with deep neck infections: a case series and review of the literature. Anesth Analg 2005;100(2):585–9.

[35] Potter J, Herford A, Ellis E. Tracheotomy versus endotracheal intubation for airway management in deep neck space infections. J Oral Maxillofac Surg 2002;60(4):349–54.

[36] Brook I. Anaerobic bacteria in upper respiratory tract and other head and neck infections. Ann Otol Rhinol Laryngol 2002;111(5 Pt 1):430–40.

[37] Thompson J, Cohen S, Reddix P. Retropharyngeal abscess in children: a retrospective and historical analysis. Laryngoscope 1988;98(6):589–92.

[38] Lee K, Tami T, Echavez M, et al. Deep neck infections in patients at risk for acquired immunodeficiency syndrome. Laryngoscope 1990;100(9):915–9.

[39] Sato K, Izumi T, Toshima M, et al. Retropharyngeal abscess due to methicillin-resistant Staphylococcus aureus in a case of acute myeloid leukemia. Intern Med 2005;44(4):346–9.

[40] Miller L, Perdreau-Remington F, Rieg G, et al. Necrotizing fasciitis caused by community-associated methicillin-resistant Staphylococcus aureus in Los Angeles. N Engl J Med 2005; 352(14):1445–53.

[41] Huang T, Tseng F, Yeh T, et al. Factors affecting the bacteriology of deep neck infection: a retrospective study of 128 patients. Acta Otolaryngol 2006;126(4):396–401.

[42] Yeow K, Liao C, Hao S. US-guided needle aspiration and catheter drainage as an alternative to open surgical drainage for uniloculated neck abscesses. J Vasc Interv Radiol 2001;12(5): 589–94.

[43] Brook I. Microbiology and management of deep facial infections and Lemierre syndrome. ORL J Otorhinolaryngol Relat Spec 2003;65(2):117–20.

[44] Lin D, Reeck J, Murr A. Internal jugular vein thrombosis and deep neck infection from intravenous drug use: management strategy. Laryngoscope 2004;114(1):56–60.

[45] Palacios E, Rojas R. Necrotizing fasciitis of the neck. Ear Nose Throat J 2006;85(10):638.

[46] Wong T. A nationwide survey of deaths from oral and maxillofacial infections: the Taiwanese experience. J Oral Maxillofac Surg 1999;57(11):1297–9.

[47] Delamaire M, Maugendre D, Moreno M, et al. Impaired leucocyte functions in diabetic patients. Diabet Med 1997;14(1):29–34.

[48] Hostetter M. Handicaps to host defense: effects of hyperglycemia on C3 and Candida albicans. Diabetes 1990;39(3):271–5.

[49] Huang T, Tseng F, Liu C, et al. Deep neck infection in diabetic patients: comparison of clinical picture and outcomes with nondiabetic patients. Otolaryngol Head Neck Surg 2005; 132(6):943–7.

[50] Lin H, Tsai C, Chen Y, et al. Influence of diabetes mellitus on deep neck infection. J Laryngol Otol 2006;120(8):650–4.

[51] Nusbaum A, Som P, Rothschild M, et al. Recurrence of a deep neck infection: a clinical indication of an underlying congenital lesion. Arch Otolaryngol Head Neck Surg 1999; 125(12):1379–82.

[52] Wang C, Ko J, Lou P. Deep neck infection as the main initial presentation of primary head and neck cancer. J Laryngol Otol 2006;120(4):305–9.

ELSEVIER
SAUNDERS

Otolaryngol Clin N Am
41 (2008) 485–496

OTOLARYNGOLOGIC
CLINICS
OF NORTH AMERICA

Diagnosis and Management of Upper Aerodigestive Tract Foreign Bodies

G. Paul Digoy, MD[a,b,*]

[a]*Department of Otorhinolaryngology, University of Oklahoma,
P.O. Box 26901, WP 1290, Oklahoma City, OK 73190, USA*
[b]*University of Oklahoma Medical Center, P.O. Box 26901,
WP 1290, Oklahoma City, OK 73190, USA*

Airway foreign bodies

Airway foreign bodies (AFBs) have remained a diagnostic challenge to health care professionals. They can become life-threatening emergencies that require immediate intervention or can go unnoticed for weeks and even months. Every effort must be made to avoid a delay in diagnosis because this may lead to a notable increase in complication rates [1]. A sudden onset of respiratory symptoms must alert the clinician to the presence of an AFB. This section presents an overview of the assessment and management of patients who have potential AFBs.

Initial patient assessment

Clinical presentation

AFBs most commonly occur in the 1- to 3-year-old child and may be related to immature dentition and a poorly coordinated swallowing mechanism. In addition, children in this age group are more likely to be active while eating and are prone to introducing various objects into their mouth. When the aspiration of a foreign body is witnessed by the caregiver, the following characteristic symptoms are often described: an early choking or gagging episode, followed by a coughing spell. As the foreign body moves distally in the airway, the symptoms often become less apparent and may even subside, creating a great diagnostic challenge because the remainder of the assessment, mainly the physical examination and radiography, can be deceptively normal [2]. Therefore, the incipient event that leads the

* 920 Stanton L. Young Boulevard, WP 1290, Oklahoma City, OK 73104.
E-mail address: paul-digoy@ouhsc.edu

0030-6665/08/$ - see front matter. Published by Elsevier Inc.
doi:10.1016/j.otc.2008.01.013

caregiver to bring the child to a health care professional can be the most important factor in the decision to proceed with a diagnostic airway endoscopy.

The classic triad of sudden onset of paroxysmal coughing, wheezing, and diminished breath sounds on the ipsilateral side is not present in all cases of foreign body aspiration. Linegar and colleagues [3] reported that among children who had a positive clinical history and a negative chest radiograph and physical examination, there was a 45% incidence of foreign bodies on airway endoscopy. They also found that in children who had a "doubtful" history, the positive yield on endoscopy was only 9.5%. Ciftci and colleagues [4] reported that a positive history was the most sensitive (91%), accurate (84%), and specific (46%) of all the diagnostic tools. Table 1 illustrates a wide range in the reported sensitivities and specificities among the three main diagnostic tools.

Peanuts, seeds, and beans are the most common aspirated matter. Peanuts and other organic objects may cause significant tissue reaction, leading to the development of granulation tissue (Fig. 1). The shape and consistency of the aspirated item can also affect the clinical picture. Relatively narrow and oval objects (such as lima beans) can change position in the airway and lead to intermittent complete airway obstruction. Grains, beans, and other vegetable matter may absorb water and can have a more rapid clinical deterioration (Fig. 2).

Physical examination

The presentation of an individual who has an AFB can range from a patient who is quiet and without discomfort to one who may exhibit signs of severe distress and impending respiratory failure. In general, the physical examination tends to have a low specificity and a variable yet higher sensitivity in predicting AFBs (see Table 1). Careful auscultation of the chest is the most critical part of the physical examination. Findings include unilateral wheezing and a discrepancy in breath sounds. Because many investigators have reported a relatively high incidence of normal physical findings (14%–45%) in patients diagnosed with an AFB on bronchoscopy [4–6], a negative physical examination should not be used to rule out the presence of an AFB. Its relatively high sensitivity, however, suggests that a positive physical examination can be a very useful tool in establishing a need for bronchoscopy.

Radiography

Plain radiographs can play an important role in the evaluation of a patient suspected of having an AFB. Although most AFBs tend to be radiolucent (~80%), certain radiograph findings can be useful in reaching a diagnosis. As the cross-sectional area of the airway increases during inspiration, air can pass beyond the foreign body. During expiration, as the cross-sectional area decreases, the air can become "trapped." Films taken during expiration can reveal hyperinflation at the ipsilateral lung (Fig. 3). This phenomenon may be less common than previously presumed [7].

Table 1
Sensitivity and specificity of diagnostic tools for AFB diagnosis

Study [Ref.]	N	History		Physical examination		Radiography	
		Sensitivity (%)	Specificity (%)	Sensitivity (%)	Specificity (%)	Sensitivity (%)	Specificity (%)
Ciftci et al, 2003 [4]	663	91	46	86	26	88	30
Zerella et al, 1998 [13][a]	293	86	82	24	64	49	n/a
Hoeve et al, 1993 [8]	115	81	33	78	37	82	44
Barrios et al, 1997 [2]	100	97	63	n/a	n/a	85	9
Metrangelo et al, 1999 [6]	87	96	76	84	12	70	63
Evan et al, 2005 [5]	98	91	45	80	60	68	71

Abbreviation: n/a, not available.
[a] Disproportionately low number of negative bronchoscopies.

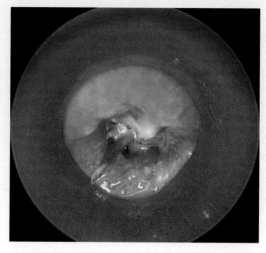

Fig. 1. Foreign body in left main-stem bronchus after delayed diagnosis. Note the purulence and granulation tissue present.

Atelectasis can be seen when the aspirated object completely obstructs the distal airway. Atelectasis and pneumonia are findings more commonly seen in the setting of delayed diagnosis (after 24 hours). Airway fluoroscopy, where available, can be a useful asset to the experienced radiologist but may have a lower sensitivity and specificity than chest radiography [5,8].

The clinician must always consider the limitations of radiography in the diagnosis of AFBs. Radiographs should not be used to rule out the presence of an AFB but used to aid in its diagnosis. Over one half of tracheal foreign bodies and 25% of bronchial foreign bodies have normal plain chest

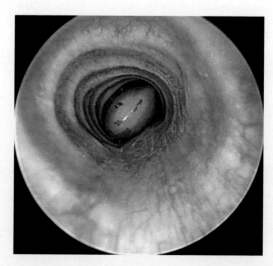

Fig. 2. Pinto bean in the tracheal airway with near-complete airway obstruction.

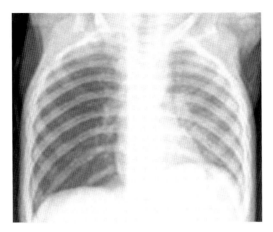

Fig. 3. Hyperinflation of the right lung secondary to a right main-stem foreign body. (*From* Kugelman A, Shaoul R, Goldsher M, et al. Persistent cough and failure to thrive: a presentation of foreign body aspiration in a child with asthma. Pediatrics 2006;177:e1057–60; with permission.)

radiographs [1]. The reported diagnostic sensitivity (49%–88%) and specificity (9%–71%) of radiographs is inconsistent and may suggest that the true yield of radiography may rely a great deal on the availability of experienced radiologists (see Table 1). Compared with history and physical examination, radiography appears to be the least sensitive in predicting bronchoscopy findings [4].

It is important to emphasize that a patient who presents with a classic history for an AFB and who may have an unpredictable or unstable airway should not be sent to a relatively unmonitored location for a radiograph. This protocol is especially relevant in younger children because the potential agitation from a chest radiograph may lead to sudden airway compromise. The use of radiography should be limited to patients who are deemed to have a stable airway and when the decision to proceed with endoscopy is in question.

Treatment recommendations

Indications for endoscopy

A delay in diagnosis is likely to increase the risk of intraoperative and postoperative complications [2,6,9–11]. To prevent a diagnostic delay, a witnessed choking event followed by a period of coughing should be considered an acceptable indication for bronchoscopy, without relying on other diagnostic tools [2,6,8,10,12]. The diagnostic tools used in the assessment of an AFB have been shown to have relatively high sensitivities, with poor and variable specificities (see Table 1). A good rule of thumb is that diagnostic bronchoscopy should be performed if any one of the three diagnostic tools (history, physical examination, or radiography) is considered positive. Furthermore, if any one of these is negative, the possibility of an AFB remains.

Many cases do not present with straightforward positive or negative findings. When the findings on physical examination, radiographs, or both are questionable, there is good evidence suggesting that both tools increase their diagnostic yield 24 hours after the event of aspiration [7]. For this reason, when the diagnosis is in question in a stable patient, the clinician can consider repeating radiography and the physical examination after a 24-hour period.

Preoperative care and anesthesia

After the diagnosis of an AFB is entertained, a patient should remain calm and monitored. The duration of fasting before endoscopy should be based on the clinician's assessment of airway stability. In acute cases of aspiration when the patient is considered unstable or potentially unstable, securing the airway should take precedence over fasting guidelines. Tomaske and colleagues [11] found that among 31 children who had symptoms of acute airway obstruction and underwent bronchoscopy without long fasting periods (<2 hours), no cases of pulmonary aspiration from gastric contents were seen. When the child is considered stable, however, the timing of endoscopy should be based on preoperative fasting guidelines and the availability of skilled personnel.

Endoscopy and foreign body removal

Extraction of the AFB requires significant skill to avoid incurring further trauma to the respiratory epithelium. The surgeon must carefully avoid pushing the foreign body distally and making the retrieval more challenging.

The skill of the anesthesiologist is also of critical importance during this procedure. It is preferable to keep the patient breathing spontaneously because this avoids significant amounts of positive pressure ventilation that may induce distal migration of the foreign body. Furthermore, during natural inspiration, the tracheal/bronchial cross-sectional area increases and may allow better access to tightly lodged foreign bodies. For spontaneous ventilation to be successful, it is imperative that the surgeon adequately anesthetize the glottis and distal airway (especially the carina) before attempting foreign body retrieval. The author's preference is to use 2% lidocaine sprayed topically to the glottis, trachea, and carina. This methodology assists the anesthesiologist in maintaining the patient's spontaneous breathing without sudden movements that can seriously complicate the procedure.

Age-appropriate equipment is crucial for preventing further trauma to the respiratory epithelium. The surgeon's familiarity with a wide assortment of laryngoscopes, bronchoscopes, and optical forceps facilitates the retrieval process and prevents unnecessary intraoperative delays. There must always be two bronchoscopes available; one that is age appropriate and one that is one size smaller.

Often the object is too large to pass through the lumen of the bronchoscope and must be removed as a single unit along with the bronchoscope and the optical forceps. When the object is sharp and facing the proximal airway, it is more safely removed when it is enclosed within the lumen of the bronchoscope [9].

Postoperative care

Chest physiotherapy can be useful in the postoperative period to help mobilize secretions and to prevent an infection. Antibiotics are not routinely used in acute cases but can play an important role in cases of delayed diagnosis (see later discussion). Generally, in the absence of complications, there are no notable interventions necessary in the postoperative setting.

Complications

Delay in diagnosis presents a significant increase in perioperative morbidity [2,6,8,10,12]. Total or near-total mainstem bronchial obstruction leads to poor alveolar aeration and subsequent shunting of pulmonary perfusion away from the affected lung. When the foreign body migrates to the contralateral side, the patient can experience abrupt respiratory decompensation [13]. This scenario is intensified in cases of delayed diagnosis because the body has more time to compensate for unilateral decrease in ventilation. Delayed diagnosis is further complicated by the development of pneumonia, atelectasis, and granulation tissue, which can lead to significant bleeding on removal of the foreign body (see Fig. 3).

Complications from bronchoscopy can also include postoperative stridor [14], bronchospasm, hypoxia, transient arrhythmias, and bradycardia. In a large case series of 3300 patients, the mortality rate was reported to be a little less than 1% [9].

Esophageal foreign bodies

Esophageal foreign bodies (EFBs) are considered less precarious than AFBs. Even so, they occur more frequently and are responsible for over 1500 deaths per year [15]. Anatomically, these foreign bodies are commonly found at the cricopharyngeus, at the crossover of the aortic arch at midesophagus, and at the lower esophageal sphincter.

Patients who have EFBs can be loosely classified into four groups: (1) pediatric patients, (2) psychiatric patients and prisoners, (3) patients who have underlying esophageal disease, and (4) edentulous adults. The largest group is the pediatric group, which corresponds to 75% to 80% of cases. Most of these children are aged 18 to 48 months [16].

Initial patient assessment

Clinical presentation

Children and adults can have very different presenting symptoms. Adults tend to intensely describe the event and acknowledge the potential for an EFB. Children can be much more vague and, in many cases (7%–35%), present with no symptoms [17–20]. When symptoms are present in children, they include irritability, poor feeding, drooling, increased work of breathing, chest pain, and coughing. Many of these symptoms can be misdiagnosed as a viral upper respiratory or gastrointestinal illnesses, and an EFB is often diagnosed incidentally on chest radiograph intended to rule out a pulmonary infiltrate [13]. If the foreign body is entrapped at the cricopharyngeus, the individual is more likely to localize the source of discomfort. Lower EFBs can have less definable symptoms such as chest pain or pressure.

Respiratory symptoms from an ingested foreign body are more common in children in whom the tracheal lumen is smaller and more compressible. These symptoms include stridor, increased work of breathing, coughing, and choking.

Physical examination

The physical examination does not play a large role in establishing an EFB diagnosis. Drooling is a concerning symptom and can be a sign of complete esophageal obstruction [21]. Symptoms of airway obstruction such as dyspnea and stridor can be seen in approximately 10% of children who have an EFB [22]. In children, the physical examination can often reveal a child who is fussy and uncooperative yet does not have specific signs or symptoms. In general, the physical examination is useful in defining the severity of the infirmity and often is not diagnostic per se.

Radiography

Unlike AFBs, the main diagnostic tool for EFBs is radiography. Foreign bodies in the esophagus are much more likely to be radiopaque. Coins are the most commonly ingested object in children (Fig. 4). A plain film should always be a part of the workup of any stable patient who has a suspected EFB. Food products are the second most common ingested object and can be confirmed on plain films when spicules of bone or cartilage are present. Anteroposterior and lateral films are required to localize the foreign body. Aanteroposterior films alone may make an AFB seem to be in the esophagus. Lateral films are also superior in identifying radiolucent foreign bodies by better identifying more subtle findings such as tracheal compression, tracheal deviation, and air trapped within the esophagus. In cases in which plain films are nondiagnostic, a barium swallow may be performed. In general, meglumine diatrizoate (Gastrografin) should not be used because it may cause severe chemical pneumonitis if aspirated.

Treatment recommendations

Indications for endoscopy

Individuals who present with symptoms of airway compromise should be taken directly to the operating room to secure the airway and retrieve the

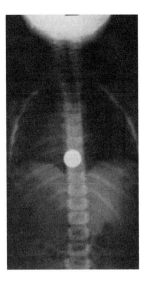

Fig. 4. A nickel in the distal esophagus of a 3-year-old child.

foreign body. The following factors should be taken into consideration in the management of less urgent cases: (1) type and location of the ingested foreign body, (2) time interval between ingestion and presentation, and (3) age of the patient. Sharp metallic objects, including pins, needles, razor blades, and nails, should all be removed endoscopically in a controlled operating room setting. Caustic ingestions such as button batteries should be considered an emergency and taken to the operating room immediately. Any delay could lead to esophageal perforation and necrosis [23].

Some authorities advocate a period of observation in stable patients who are not in respiratory distress, do not have significant discomfort, and who do not have known esophageal anomalies [17–19,24,25]. The goal of observation is spontaneous passage of the foreign body into the stomach. This approach is not indicated in a patient who presents more than 24 hours after ingestion or who has pooling and intolerance of oral secretions. The rate of spontaneous passage is related to the anatomic location of the foreign body in the esophagus. Waltzman and colleagues [26] reported that coins located in the upper third, middle third, and lower third of the esophagus spontaneously pass to the stomach 14%, 43%, and 67% of the time, respectively. In this prospective study, half of the patients who spontaneously passed the ingested coins did so after 6 hours of observation; the other half by 19 hours. Male gender is also a significant predictor of spontaneous passage. Coin size did not appear to play a major role [26]. Some studies have suggested that outpatient observation after coin ingestion is safe in the stable and relatively asymptomatic child [17–19]. The period of observation should not be longer than 24 hours; a period of 8 to 16 hours is generally considered acceptable in asymptomatic children who have esophageal coins.

Endoscopy and foreign body removal

Esophagoscopy is considered a safe procedure with an excellent foreign body retrieval rate. When there is any evidence of respiratory difficulty, esophagoscopy should be performed in the operating room after a secure airway is achieved. The choice of flexible versus rigid esophagoscopy should be based on the experience of the endoscopist and the equipment available. Some centers reserve rigid esophagoscopy for foreign bodies above the cricopharyngeus, and flexible esophagoscopy for foreign bodies in the lower esophagus. Both methods are safe and effective in the hands of a well-trained and experienced endoscopist [27,28]. A benefit of flexible esophagoscopy is that it can be done in an endoscopy suite under conscious sedation, whereas rigid esophagoscopy usually requires general anesthesia in the operating room. Rigid endoscopy, however, accommodates a larger variety of grasping forceps and allows for superior optics and magnification. An essential benefit of either method is its ability to examine the esophageal wall after the object is removed.

Alternative methods of foreign body removal

Balloon catheter extraction of EFBs is receiving increasing attention as a cost-effective alternative to endoscopy in select patients [29–31]. Indications include the presence of a single, smooth, and radiopaque foreign body. There should be no history of esophageal disease or surgery. Any evidence of respiratory difficulty is considered an absolute contraindication for this technique. Ingestion must have taken place less than 72 hours before the procedure. Endoscopic backup should always be available. Due to the inherent risk for airway complications, resuscitation equipment and personnel familiar with advanced airway management must be present.

This procedure is performed by first placing the patient in head-down position. The clinician passes a catheter nasally or orally under fluoroscopic guidance past the foreign body. The balloon catheter is inflated with a radioopaque solution and is slowly removed under fluoroscopic guidance. Mild complications have included epistaxis and foreign body dislodgement into the nose. Cases of laryngospasm, hypoxia, and hyperpyrexia have also been reported.

Advocates for this method report cost savings of over $1800 per patient [32], low complication rates [30,31,33], and high success rates (85%–100%) [30,31,34,35]; however, proponents fail to acknowledge the potentially inhumane side of this technique when restraining devices are used in nonsedated children. In addition, the benefit of endoscopically examining the esophageal mucosa before and after foreign body retrieval should be taken into consideration, especially when the foreign body is present for over 24 hours. The greatest concern is with centers that employ this technique without adequate equipment and personnel trained in airway management. For this procedure to gain nationwide acceptance, safety standards should be established that make certain of the adequacy of technical training and ensure that airway safety measures are always in place.

Complications

Similar to AFBs, EFBs have a greater complication rate when the diagnosis is delayed [36]. The relative risk for complications has been found to be greater than 1 when duration of lodgment is longer than 24 hours and increases to 6.83 for duration of lodgment longer than 72 hours [10]. Esophageal injuries can range from mild abrasions or lacerations to necrosis, perforation, and vascular injuries. The consequence of the initial insult may not manifest itself for days and even weeks after the foreign body is removed. Serious complications such as mediastinitis, pneumothorax, tracheoesophageal fistula, and vascular injuries (aorta-esophageal fistula) can be life threatening. Early diagnosis and a safe retrieval method is the key to avoiding complications.

References

[1] Mu L, He P, Sun D. The causes and complications of late diagnosis of foreign body aspiration in children. Report of 210 cases. Arch Otolaryngol Head Neck Surg 1991;117(8):876–9.

[2] Barrios Fontoba JE, Gutierrez C, Lluna J, et al. Bronchial foreign body: should bronchoscopy be performed in all patients with a choking crisis? Pediatr Surg Int 1997;12(2–3):118–20.

[3] Linegar AG, von Oppell UO, Hegemann S, et al. Tracheobronchial foreign bodies. Experience at Red Cross Children's Hospital, 1985–1990. S Afr Med J 1992;82(3).164–7.

[4] Ciftci AO, Bingol-Kololu M, Senocak ME, et al. Bronchoscopy for evaluation of foreign body aspiration in children. J Pediatr Surg 2003;38(8):1170–6.

[5] Even L, Heno N, Talmon Y, et al. Diagnostic evaluation of foreign body aspiration in children: a prospective study [erratum appears in J Pediatr Surg. 2005 Nov;40(11):1815 Note: Lea, Even [corrected to Even, Lea]; Nawaf, Heno [corrected to Heno, Nawaf]; Yoav, Talmon [corrected to Talmon, Yoav]; Elvin, Samet [corrected to Samet, Elvin]; Ze'ev, Zonis [corrected to Zonis, Ze'ev]; Amir, Kugelman [corrected to Kugelman, Amir]. J Pediatr Surg 2005;40(7):1122–7.

[6] Metrangelo S, Monetti C, Meneghini L, et al. Eight years' experience with foreign-body aspiration in children: what is really important for a timely diagnosis? J Pediatr Surg 1999; 34(8):1229–31.

[7] Tokar B, Ozkan R, Ilhan H. Tracheobronchial foreign bodies in children: importance of accurate history and plain chest radiography in delayed presentation. Clin Radiol 2004;59(7): 609–15.

[8] Hoeve LJ, Rombout J, Pot DJ. Foreign body aspiration in children. The diagnostic value of signs, symptoms and pre-operative examination. Clin Otolaryngol Allied Sci 1993;18(1): 55–7.

[9] Sersar SI, Rizk WH, Bilal M, et al. Inhaled foreign bodies: presentation, management and value of history and plain chest radiography in delayed presentation. Otolaryngol Head Neck Surg 2006;134(1):92–9.

[10] Tokar B, Cevik AA, Ilhan H. Ingested gastrointestinal foreign bodies: predisposing factors for complications in children having surgical or endoscopic removal. Pediatr Surg Int 2007; 23(2):135–9.

[11] Tomaske M, Gerber AC, Weiss M. Anesthesia and periinterventional morbidity of rigid bronchoscopy for tracheobronchial foreign body diagnosis and removal. Paediatr Anaesth 2006;16(2):123–9.

[12] Wolach B, Raz A, Weinberg J, et al. Aspirated foreign bodies in the respiratory tract of children: eleven years experience with 127 patients. Int J Pediatr Otorhinolaryngol 1994;30(1): 1–10.

[13] Gibson. Aerodigestive tract foreign bodies. In: Cotton RT, Meyer CM III, editors. Practical Pediatric Otolaryngology. p. 561.
[14] Zerella JT, Dimler M, McGill LC, et al. Foreign body aspiration in children: value of radiography and complications of bronchoscopy. J Pediatr Surg 1998;33(11):1651–4.
[15] Uyemura MC. Foreign body ingestion in children [erratum appears in Am Fam Physician. 2006 Apr 15;73(8):1332]; [summary for patients in Am Fam Physician. 2005 Jul 15;72(2):292; PMID: 16050453]. [Review] [11 refs]. Am Fam Physician 2005;72(2):287–91.
[16] Stack LB, Munter DW. Foreign bodies in the gastrointestinal tract [review] [88 refs]. Emerg Med Clin North Am 1996;14(3):493–521.
[17] Conners GP, Chamberlain JM, Ochsenschlager DW. Symptoms and spontaneous passage of esophageal coins [see comment]. Arch Pediatr Adolesc Med 1995;149(1):36–9.
[18] Conners GP, Chamberlain JM, Ochsenschlager DW. Conservative management of pediatric distal esophageal coins. J Emerg Med 1996;14(6):723–6.
[19] Conners GP, Cobaugh DJ, Feinberg R, et al. Home observation for asymptomatic coin ingestion: acceptance and outcomes. The New York State Poison Control Center Coin Ingestion Study Group. Acad Emerg Med 1999;6(3):213–7.
[20] Hodge D III, Tecklenburg F, Fleisher G. Coin ingestion: does every child need a radiograph? Ann Emerg Med 1985;14(5):443–6.
[21] Lyons MF, Tsuchida AM. Foreign bodies of the gastrointestinal tract [review] [84 refs]. Med Clin North Am 1993;77(5):1101–14.
[22] Crysdale WS, Sendi KS, Yoo J. Esophageal foreign bodies in children. 15-year review of 484 cases. Ann Otol Rhinol Laryngol 1991;100(4 Pt 1):320–4.
[23] Litovitz T, Schmitz BF. Ingestion of cylindrical and button batteries: an analysis of 2382 cases [see comment]. Pediatrics 1992;89(4 Pt 2):747–57.
[24] Gracia C, Frey CF, Bodai BI. Diagnosis and management of ingested foreign bodies: a ten-year experience. Ann Emerg Med 1984;13(1):30–4.
[25] Soprano JV, Fleisher GR, Mandl KD. The spontaneous passage of esophageal coins in children. Arch Pediatr Adolesc Med 1999;153(10):1073–6.
[26] Waltzman ML, Baskin M, Wypij D, et al. A randomized clinical trial of the management of esophageal coins in children [see comment]. Pediatrics 2005;116(3):614–9.
[27] Hsu W, Sheen T, Lin C, et al. Clinical experiences of removing foreign bodies in the airway and esophagus with a rigid endoscope: a series of 3217 cases from 1970 to 1996. Otolaryngol Head Neck Surg 2000;122(3):450–4.
[28] Li ZS, Sun ZX, Zou DW, et al. Endoscopic management of foreign bodies in the upper-GI tract: experience with 1088 cases in China [see comment]. Gastrointest Endosc 2006;64(4):485–92.
[29] Harned RK, Strain JD, Hay TC, et al. Esophageal foreign bodies: safety and efficacy of Foley catheter extraction of coins. AJR Am J Roentgenol 1997;168(2):443–6.
[30] Little DC, Shah SR, St Peter SD, et al. Esophageal foreign bodies in the pediatric population: our first 500 cases. J Pediatr Surg 2006;41(5):914–8.
[31] Morrow SE, Bickler SW, Kennedy AP, et al. Balloon extraction of esophageal foreign bodies in children [see comment]. J Pediatr Surg 1998;33(2):266–70.
[32] Kelley JE, Leech MH, Carr MG. A safe and cost-effective protocol for the management of esophageal coins in children. J Pediatr Surg 1993;28(7):898–900.
[33] Schunk JE, Harrison AM, Corneli HM, et al. Fluoroscopic Foley catheter removal of esophageal foreign bodies in children: experience with 415 episodes [see comment]. Pediatrics 1994; 94(5):709–14.
[34] Campbell JB, Davis WS. Catheter technique for extraction of blunt esophageal foreign bodies. Radiology 1973;108(2):438–40.
[35] Mariani PJ, Wagner DK. Foley catheter extraction of blunt esophageal foreign bodies. J Emerg Med 1986;4(4):301–6.
[36] Chaikhouni A, Kratz JM, Crawford FA. Foreign bodies of the esophagus. Am Surg 1985; 51(4):173–9.

ELSEVIER
SAUNDERS

Otolaryngol Clin N Am
41 (2008) 497–524

OTOLARYNGOLOGIC
CLINICS
OF NORTH AMERICA

Invasive Fungal Sinusitis and Complications of Rhinosinusitis

Victoria A. Epstein, MD, Robert C. Kern, MD*

*Department of Otolaryngology Head and Neck Surgery, Feinberg School of Medicine,
Northwestern University, 303 East Chicago Avenue, Searle Building 12-561,
Chicago, IL 60611, USA*

Invasive fungal sinusitis

Invasive fungal sinusitis is one of the most challenging forms of sinonasal pathology to manage, most commonly presenting in immunocompromised individuals. Diagnosis of invasive fungal sinusitis requires histopathologic evidence of fungi invading nasal tissue: hyphal forms within the sinus mucosa, submucosa, blood vessels, or bone [1]. Invasive fungal sinusitis has been subclassified into three distinct forms: acute fulminant invasive fungal sinusitis (AFIFS), chronic invasive fungal sinusitis, and granulomatous invasive fungal sinusitis [1–3]. The focus of this article is on the acute fulminant form of invasive rhinosinusitis, the most common subtype in the United States. Failure to diagnose and treat this entity promptly usually results in rapid progression and death.

AFIFS results from the rapid spread of fungi from the nasal and sinus mucosa by way of vascular invasion into the orbit, vessels, and parenchyma of the brain. The time course of less than 4 weeks' duration separates acute from chronic disease [4]. Patients typically have ailments associated with impaired neutrophil function (hematologic malignancies, aplastic anemia, hemochromatosis, insulin-dependent diabetes, AIDS, organ transplantation) or are undergoing iatrogenic immunosuppression with systemic steroids or chemotherapeutic agents [1–5]. Although rare, cases of AFIFS in otherwise healthy individuals have been documented in the literature [5–7].

* Corresponding author. Department of Otolaryngology – Head and Neck Surgery, Feinberg School of Medicine, Northwestern University, 303 East Chicago Avenue, Searle Building 12-561, Chicago, IL 60611.

E-mail address: r-kern@northwestern.edu (R.C. Kern).

0030-6665/08/$ - see front matter © 2008 Elsevier Inc. All rights reserved.
doi:10.1016/j.otc.2008.01.001   *oto.theclinics.com*

Diagnosis

Several studies have investigated the signs and symptoms of AFIFS to determine the subset of patients who require a more aggressive diagnostic investigation. In the immunocompromised patient population, the presence of fever of unknown origin after 48 hours of appropriate broad-spectrum intravenous antibiotic or the presence of localizing sinonasal symptoms should prompt imaging studies and nasal endoscopy [4,5,8]. The physical findings in AFIFS can be subtle, but the most consistent finding is an alteration in the appearance of the nasal mucosa. Mucosal discoloration can be variable, and may be gray, green, white, or black. Discoloration, granulation, and ulceration typically replace the normal pale-pink mucosa. White discoloration indicates tissue ischemia secondary to angiocentric invasion, whereas black discoloration is a late finding of tissue necrosis. In a series by Gillespie and colleagues [9], mucosal abnormalities were seen most commonly on the middle turbinate, followed by the septum, palate, and inferior turbinate. Anesthetic regions of the face or oral cavity are features of early invasive process and may precede the development of objective changes in the mucosa. Decreased nasal mucosal bleeding or sensation should also be noted because they may be signs of fungal invasion.

Intraoperative nasal endoscopic examination may be the most informative test for possible fungal involvement in pediatric patients who have severe neutropenia (absolute neutrophil count 600 cells/μL or fewer), persistent fevers, or localizing sinus symptoms. Park and colleagues [8] discovered that bedside endoscopic findings did not correlate with intraoperative endoscopy because of a large amount of debris in the nasal cavity that was not removed during bedside examinations and the relative noncompliance of the pediatric patients. Examination under general anesthesia was recommended for nasal endoscopic examination and directed biopsies of suspicious lesions, the middle and inferior turbinate.

CT of paranasal sinuses is usually obtained during the workup of immunocompromised patients who have fever or sinonasal symptoms, usually before evaluation by an otolaryngologist. Fine-cut (2-mm) slices in the axial and coronal planes should be obtained in high-risk patients. Intravenous contrast is used if intracranial or intraorbital extension is suspected, but it is not necessary for most initial evaluations. Severe unilateral thickening of the nasal cavity mucosa has been shown to be the most consistent finding on CT, suggestive of underlying invasive fungal sinusitis [10]. It has also been suggested that infiltration of the periantral fat planes (Fig. 1) may represent the earliest imaging evidence of AFIFS [11]. Although the diagnosis of AFIFS cannot be made on the basis of imaging, CT scans are helpful in defining individual variations in sinus architecture and possible periorbital and intracranial spread. MRI is superior to CT in delineating the intracranial extent of the disease and it may have a role in evaluating patients who demonstrate signs of intracranial invasion: mental status changes, orbital apex syndrome, seizure, or stroke.

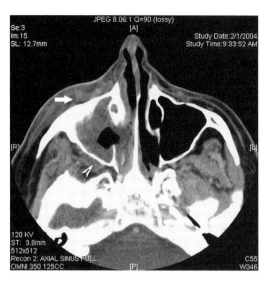

Fig. 1. Axial contrast-enhanced CT demonstrating right maxillary sinus opacification with soft tissue infiltration of the right posterior periantral fat plane (*arrowhead*) and premaxillary soft tissue (*white arrow*) in a diabetic patient with AFIFS (Rhizopus). (*Courtesy of* Achilles Karagianis, MD, Chicago, IL.)

Diagnosis of AFIFS incorporates clinical suspicion with culture and microscopic examination of the specimens. Because prompt diagnosis is essential, the potassium hydroxide–calcofluor white method can be used immediately on culture aspirate material. This highly sensitive technique uses potassium hydroxide to dissolve human material, and an optic brightener (calcofluor white) that binds to the cell wall of the hyphae. Fungal cell walls, including septations, fluoresce when viewed using a fluorescence microscope [12]. The fungal cultures may take days to weeks to grow but may be needed for antifungal susceptibility testing. Proper speciation also provides important clinical data, because certain species, such as *Pseudallescheria boydii*, do not respond to amphotericin. Histopathologic evaluation of the suspected tissue, however, is typically the most critical to making the diagnosis. Permanent section with the Gomori-methenamine-silver stain uses deposition of silver onto the fungal cell wall, and, because it can detect even a single cell, it undoubtedly is the most sensitive of the commonly used histologic stains. No histologic specimen should be considered to be negative for fungus unless a silver stain has been performed [12]. Fungal disease is determined to be invasive if it meets the following criteria: (1) hyphal forms within the submucosa, with or without angiocentric invasion and (2) tissue necrosis with minimal host inflammatory cell infiltration [2]. Frozen section allows for a timely diagnosis, and, if positive, appropriate antifungal therapy and extended surgical resection can be initiated without delay. Neither frozen section nor special stains will definitely distinguish among fungal species, but this distinction can generally be made on permanent histopath-ologic sections. *Mucormycosis* fungal elements are broad, ribbon-like, irreg-ular, and rarely septated, whereas the *Aspergillus* sp demonstrate more narrow hyphae with regular septations and 45° branching [4,5]. *Aspergillus* sp can be angioinvasive, but it is not the obliterative invasion seen with *mucormycosis*.

Treatment and prognosis

The treatment of AFIFS requires reversal of the underlying predisposing condition, surgical debridement, and appropriate systemic antifungal ther-apy. Treatment of diabetic ketoacidosis or correction of neutropenia can be initiated concurrently with systemic antifungals. In transplant patients, or those who have hematologic malignancies, white blood cell transfusions and administration of granulocyte colony–stimulating factor to increase an absolute neutrophil count to above $1000/mm^3$ have been shown to improve survival [5,13,14].

Medical antifungal therapy for most patients who have AFIFS consists of systemic amphotericin B at intravenous doses of 0.25 to 1.0 mg/kg/d to a to-tal dose of 2 to 4 g over six to eight weeks. The use of amphotericin B is lim-ited in some patients secondary to renal toxicity, and they may be candidates for liposomal amphotericin B at a concentration of 3 to 5 mg/kg/d. Liposo-mal amphotericin, secondary to high cost, is reserved for a clinically proven fungal infection in an immunocompromised host with an elevated serum creatinine (>2.5 mg/dL) or progression of fungal disease while on maximum dosage of standard amphotericin. Voriconazole, approved by the Food and Drug Administration in 2002, is more effective than amphotericin B for invasive aspergillus [15].

Antifungals alone are not sufficient in the treatment of invasive fungal sinusitis. Early aggressive endoscopic sinonasal debridement should be per-formed on all patients who have biopsy-proven disease or on any patient suspected of having fungal invasion. Radical resections (radical maxillec-tomy, craniofacial resection, and orbital exenteration) to remove disease outside the sinonasal cavity rarely achieve negative margins or improve long-term survival [9,16]. Endoscopic sinus debridement slows the progres-sion of the disease, reduces the fungal load, and provides a specimen for culture and histopathologic diagnosis [5]. Debridement of the involved sinuses or structures is extended until clear bleeding margins are exposed. Hemorrhage in thrombocytopenic patients can be reduced if the platelet count is greater than $60 \times 10^9/L$. A second-look procedure should be sched-uled within 48 to 72 hours if residual disease in the sinonasal cavity is suspected. Follow-up consists of weekly rigid nasal endoscopy until reversal of neutropenia, and should be once a month for 6 months thereafter [5].

Although earlier studies have cited the mortality for AFIFS to be as high as 50% to 80%, more recent series have demonstrated a mortality rate of less than 20% [14]. However, a mortality rate approaching 100% has been demonstrated in patients who have symptomatic intracranial involvement [9,16,17]. Thus, patients who have orbital apex involvement or intracranial spread are less likely to respond to radical surgery, and should be appropriately counseled when a radical surgical procedure is considered [5]. Identification of the fungal organism can also be an important predictor of survival. The overall mortality of patients infected with Mucor (29%) is higher than in those infected with aspergillus (11%), regardless of the patient's underlying condition [14]. The survival rates in those with invasive mucormycosis reflect the variance in the ability to reverse the underlying predisposing cause [18]. Neutropenic patients who respond to granulocyte colony–stimulating factor are more likely to become disease survivors; this subset of patients is more likely to have disease limited to the sinonasal cavity, which is also more amenable to limited resection [9]. In a large retrospective review by Parikh [14], the overall mortality rate directly as a result of invasive fungal sinusitis was found to be 18%. When examining each specific disease subgroup, the mortality rate from invasive fungal sinusitis among diabetic patients (40%) was significantly higher than in patients who had hematologic malignancy (11%), chronic steroid users (33%), and solid organ transplant patients (0%). This disparity can be due to a greater incidence of *Mucor* over *Aspergillus* affecting diabetics and a delay in diagnosis resulting in more advanced disease at presentation in this subgroup of patients [14].

Complications of rhinosinusitis

Rhinosinusitis has become one of the most common chronic illnesses in the United States, affecting one in eight persons [19]. Complications of rhinosinusitis range from relatively benign to potentially fatal and are divided into three categories: local, orbital, and intracranial.

Local complications

Mucocele
Paranasal sinus mucoceles are chronic, cystic lesions that are lined with pseudostratified or low-columnar epithelium containing occasional goblet cells. These are slowly concentrically expanding lesions, frequently requiring more than 10 years to become symptomatic. Although the exact pathophysiologic mechanisms are still uncertain, mucoceles are generally classified as primary or secondary [20]. Primary mucoceles (also called mucus retention cysts) develop secondary to blockage of the duct of a minor salivary gland within the lining of the paranasal sinus, primarily in the maxillary sinus, and are not discussed further here.

A secondary mucocele results from obstruction of a sinus ostium caused by the obstructive complications of chronic rhinosinusitis, polyposis, trauma, surgery, or tumor. The sinuses most commonly involved (in

decreasing order of frequency) are the frontal sinus, ethmoid sinuses, maxillary sinus, and sphenoid sinus [21,22]. Headache and diminished vision
constitute the most common presenting symptoms of sphenoid sinus mucocele [23,24]. The most common clinically significant mucocele originates in
the frontal sinus where sinusitis in a chronic state can predispose to slow
formation of a mucocele over the course of many years [25].

Diagnosis. Frontal headache and proptosis are the most common presenting complaints of patients who have frontal mucocele, with displacement
of the globe in a downward and outward direction. Deep nasal or periorbital
pain may occur. In contrast to acute or chronic sinusitis, nasal obstruction
and rhinorrhea are unusual findings [20,26]. Although the diagnosis may be
suggested by the clinical presentation, past medical history, or physical
examination, radiographic imaging is necessary for accurate analysis of
the regional anatomy and the extent of the lesion. On CT scan, mucoceles
appear as hypodense, nonenhancing masses that fill and expand the sinus
cavity. The typical mucocele contents have low density and do not enhance.
As the mucus becomes more inspissated, the density may increase. On MRI,
the signal intensity of the mucocele varies with its protein content and the
degree of hydration (Fig. 2). After injection of gadolinium contrast, on
T1-weighted image with fat suppression, the mucocele shows no enhancement, with some enhancement of the mucosa along the margin of the

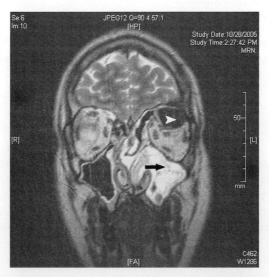

Fig. 2. MRI T2-weighted coronal image before contrast showing left frontal (*arrowhead*) and
left maxillary (*black arrow*) mucoceles. The left frontal sinus mucocele has a different T2 signal
(hypointense) compared with the left maxillary sinus (hyperintense) because of more inspissated
secretions (less water content). (*Courtesy of* Achilles Karagianis, MD, Chicago, IL.)

mucocele. This finding can help rule out solid tumors, which show significant enhancement [22,27].

Treatment. Traditional management of mucoceles emphasized the need for complete removal of the lining to achieve a cure, usually involving an open surgical approach. More recently, transnasal endoscopic techniques have essentially replaced the earlier methodology for most mucoceles. Endoscopic marsupialization of mucoceles, rather than complete removal, as a treatment concept, relies on the ability of the sinus mucosa to return to a normal or near-normal condition [28,29].

Frontal sinus mucoceles differ from similar lesions of other sinuses in that the frontal outflow tract is usually narrower and less accessible for conventional intranasal surgery. The osteoplastic flap with fat obliteration has been the gold standard against which other frontal sinus procedures have been compared. More recently, endoscopic drainage and marsupialization techniques have largely replaced the osteoplastic flap for the management of frontal mucoceles, with recurrence rates at, or close to, 0% [26,30–33]. Har-el [32] treated 66 frontal and frontoethmoidal mucoceles endoscopically and reported a recurrence rate of 0.9%. For frontal sinus mucoceles, a minimum Draf II procedure was performed and most large mucoceles were managed with a Draf III, also termed the endoscopic modified Lothrop procedure (EMLP). A retrospective study [33] evaluated the efficacy of EMLP for complicated frontal mucoceles treated over a 4-year period (1998–2002). Twenty-one patients underwent the EMLP and, at a median follow-up of 16 months, all patients had a patent mucocele opening and had improvement in symptoms and signs. Although excellent results have been confirmed, given the nature of mucoceles, long-term results (5–10 year follow-ups) are needed before endoscopic drainage of these lesions can be validated completely. Furthermore, although mucoceles of paranasal sinuses are increasingly treated by endoscopic surgery, external approaches with or without obliteration of the sinus occasionally remain useful as tools in the treatment of this disease.

Osteomyelitis and Pott's puffy tumor

The frontal sinus is the most common sinus involved with osteomyelitis; osteomyelitis of other sinuses is rare [34]. Pott's puffy tumor (PPT), first described by Sir Percivall Pott in 1775, is a subperiosteal abscess (SPA) of the frontal bone that appears as a localized swelling of the overlying region of the forehead associated with frontal osteomyelitis [35]. PPT can result from acute and chronic frontal sinusitis and has become an uncommon entity since the introduction of antibiotics. Although the association of epidural purulent collections with PPT is well recognized, other intracranial abnormalities, such as subdural empyema and intracerebral abscess, have also been described.

The sinus mucosa, marrow cavity, and frontal bone share common venous drainage through the valveless diploic veins. The spread of infection from the frontal sinuses into the frontal bone causes inflammation in the diploic system, with local suppuration, that propagates to the Haversian system of the inner and outer tables of the skull and causes localized demineralization and necrosis. This process then leads to perforation of the anterior table of the frontal sinus, resulting in the subperiosteal pus collection and formation of granulation tissue known as PPT. The involvement of the venous structures explains the development of epidural abscess in cases where the posterior wall of the frontal sinus is intact, or the presence of subdural empyema without epidural abscess or dural violation [36–40].

The most common causative organisms are *Staphylococcus aureus*, non-enterococcal *streptococcus*, and oral anaerobes. Cultures from patients who have PTT often reveal polymicrobial involvement. When intracranial complications occur, anaerobes such as *Fusobacterium*, *Bacteroides*, and anaerobic *Streptococci* are the predominant pathogens [41,42]. It has been suggested that the reason why these organisms are common in frontal sinusitis, although uncommon in diseases affecting other sinuses, is the relatively lower oxygen concentration in the frontal sinus [37].

Diagnosis. The presenting symptoms of osteomyelitis and PPT include headache, photophobia, swelling of the forehead, purulent and nonpurulent rhinorrhea, and fever. Fluctuant and tender erythematous swelling of the scalp at the midforehead is a typical sign [36,37,43]. In complicated cases with intracranial abscesses, headache is almost always present, in addition to signs of increased intracranial pressure (nausea, vomiting, lethargy) and focal neurologic deficits [36,37].

CT (Fig. 3) is the diagnostic modality of choice for PPT, but MRI is the gold standard for the diagnosis of any intracranial complication. On CT with contrast, SPA will be visualized as a hypodense collection of fluid external to the frontal bone with an enhancing rim that represents the thickened, displaced periosteum; this finding corresponds to the clinically palpable PPT [44].

Treatment. Surgical intervention is the treatment of choice for PPT. Treatment should include intravenous administration of broad-spectrum antibiotics followed by evacuation of the SPA and removal of the osteomyelitic bone up to the margins of normal bone. Consistent with the literature on osteomyelitis in long bones, antibiotic therapy for a minimum of 6 weeks is recommended. Anticonvulsants are used in patients who have intradural infection [43].

Frontal sinusitis can be addressed through endoscopic frontal sinusotomy and through external approaches such as frontal trephination. Functional endoscopic sinus surgery has been advocated for the treatment of acute complicated sinusitis [45,46], and endoscopic frontal sinusotomy has

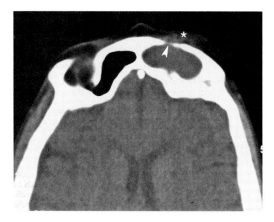

Fig. 3. Axial CT scan with soft tissue window revealing destruction of the anterior table of the frontal sinus (*arrowhead*) with inflammation extending into the forehead soft tissues (*asterisk*). (*Courtesy of* Achilles Karagianis, MD, Chicago, IL.)

the advantage of avoiding facial scars, preserving the bony superstructure of the frontal sinus infundibulum, and preserving a greater amount of mucosa than an external approach [47]. However, the risk of major complications varies between 1% and 2% and may increase when the surgery is performed on acutely inflamed sinuses, when the increased vascularity and consequent hemorrhage may obscure the operative field [48]. Frontal trephination is a relatively simple and effective procedure, and it can be a mainstay of treatment for complicated sinusitis requiring immediate surgical treatment. Mortimore and Wormald [49] found that 80% of patients who had complicated sinusitis undergoing frontal sinus trephine, irrigations, and drainage of purulence did not require further surgery. If definitive surgery is still required after the frontal sinus trephine, it can be performed at a later date under more advantageous conditions.

Orbital complications

The spread of infection from the paranasal sinuses to the orbit represents the most common site of extension of rhinosinusitis. Ethmoid sinusitis can extend through the thin lamina papyracea or through congenital, surgical, or traumatic dehiscences in the medial or superior walls. The infections may also spread into the orbit through the anterior and posterior ethmoid neurovascular foramina and the valveless veins (communicating between the nose, paranasal sinuses, pterygoid plexus, and the orbit). Although frontal sinusitis alone rarely causes orbital complications, communication from the frontal sinus to the orbit may occur in three sites of dehiscence in the frontal bone: behind the trochlear fossa, behind the supraorbital notch, and at the junction of the middle and outer thirds of the sinus floor [50]. Sinusitis-related orbital infection is the most common cause of unilateral proptosis in children and the third leading cause in adults, behind Graves' orbitopathy and pseudotumor [51]. Children appear to be more prone to orbital complications, probably secondary to the high incidence of acute rhinosinusitis in the pediatric population. Based on the anatomy and the presumed pathogenesis of orbital infections, Chandler [52] classified the orbital complications into five groups, as shown in Table 1.

Orbital complications are most commonly the result of *Streptococcus* sp, anaerobic micro-organisms, *Staphylococcus* sp, and other organisms associated with sinusitis, including gram-negative bacilli. Although a broad range of *Streptococcus* is implicated in rhinosinusitis and its complications, recent series have specifically identified *Streptococcus milleri* as an isolate in orbital and intracranial complications [53].

Inflammatory edema

Preseptal cellulitis describes infection limited to the skin and subcutaneous tissues of the eyelid anterior to the orbital septum. It is the most common and least severe complication, and is responsible for approximately 70% of all orbital complications of sinusitis [25]. Preseptal cellulitis is more common than orbital cellulitis, especially in children, and results from impeded venous and lymphatic drainage from the obstructed sinus.

Diagnosis. Examination of a patient who has preseptal cellulitis will reveal eyelid swelling, erythema, and tenderness. Visual acuity, pupillary reaction, extraocular motility, and intraocular pressure are normal. CT is usually unnecessary in patients who have preseptal infections, but, if done, would reveal a diffuse increase in density and thickening of the lid and conjunctiva [54]. CT is mandatory when intracranial complications are suspected or when signs or symptoms of postseptal inflammation (findings of proptosis, gaze restriction, or changes in visual acuity) progress in 24 to 48 hours despite therapy [55].

Table 1
Chandler's classification of orbital infection

I. Inflammatory edema (preseptal)	Lid edema, no limitation in ocular movement or visual change
II. Orbital cellulitis (postseptal)	Diffuse orbital infection and inflammation without abscess formation
III. Subperiosteal abscess	Collection of pus between medial periosteum and lamina papyracea, impaired extraocular movement
IV. Orbital abscess	Discrete pus collection in orbital tissues, proptosis and chemosis with ophthalmoplegia and decreased vision
V. Cavernous sinus thrombosis	Bilateral eye findings and worsening of all other previously described eye findings

Treatment. The management of preseptal cellulitis should include broad-spectrum oral antibiotics, head elevation, warm packs, and management of the underlying cause. Although intravenous antibiotics were standard care for preseptal cellulitis in children before the introduction of the *Haemophilus influenzae* type B (Hib) vaccination in 1985, oral broad-spectrum antibiotics are now often appropriate for mild cases and when good follow-up is ensured [56]. Controversy still remains as to whether these patients should be admitted for intravenous antibiotics and close examination, especially children under 3 years of age. A nasal decongestant, either topical or oral, mucolytics, and saline irrigations may help promote sinus drainage.

Orbital cellulitis

Orbital cellulitis defines an infectious process that occurs within the orbit proper, behind the orbital septum, and within the bony walls of the orbit. The orbital contents show diffuse edema with inflammatory cells and fluid, without distinct abscess formation. The swelling of orbital contents occurs when an increase in sinus venous pressure is transmitted to the orbital vasculature, resulting in transudation and leakage through the vessel walls [54].

Diagnosis. Clinically, the patient has eyelid edema, mild proptosis, and chemosis. Orbital pain is present in 85% of patients [57]. In severe cases, motility may be limited; however, visual acuity is not impaired. When orbital cellulitis is suspected, ophthalmologic consultation should be obtained to assess visual acuity, pupillary reaction, confrontation visual fields, color vision, extraocular motility, proptosis, globe displacement, resistance to globe retropulsion, intraocular pressure, and optic nerve appearance [55]. Orbital imaging should be obtained in all patients suspected of having orbital cellulitis. Axial and coronal views of the orbits and sinuses with contrast should be obtained in soft tissue and bone windows. CT with contrast (Fig. 4) will show some enhancement of edematous orbital fatty reticulum and adjacent tissues. The involvement is maximal in the extraconal fat directly adjacent to the most severely affected sinus. Although proptosis is usually present, suggestive of more diffuse involvement, intraconal fat may be radiographically normal. Other findings include eyelid swelling, which is uniformly present, and enlargement and contrast enhancement of the adjacent rectus muscle, which is present in some cases [54].

Treatment. After initial evaluation by an ophthalmologist, orbital cellulitis patient should have daily assessments of visual acuity and color vision, pupillary reaction, and extraocular motility. Early treatment should include intravenous antibiotics and imaging to determine which orbital and associated sites are involved. Antibiotic failure is indicated by progression of vision loss, persistent fever after 36 hours of antibiotic treatment, clinical deterioration after 48 hours of antibiotics, or failure to improve within

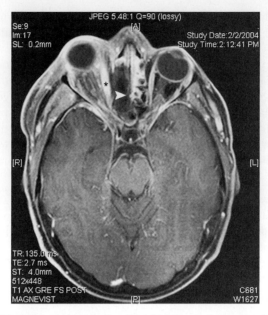

Fig. 4. Enhanced fat-suppressed axial T1-weighted MRI revealing right orbital cellulitis with right-sided anterior ethmoid sinusitis (*arrowhead*) and proptosis and thickening of the right medial rectus (*asterisk*). (*Courtesy of* Achilles Karagianis, MD, Chicago, IL.)

72 hours of antibiotic treatment [58]. Surgical drainage is recommended when one of five circumstances is present [55]:

- CT evidence of abscess formation
- Visual acuity of 20/60 (or worse) on initial evaluation
- Severe orbital complications (eg, blindness or an afferent pupillary reflex) on initial evaluation
- Progression of orbital signs and symptoms despite therapy
- Lack of improvement within 48 hours despite medical therapy

Surgical treatment should include adequate drainage of the infected sinuses.

Subperiosteal abscess

SPA is most commonly located in the superomedial or inferomedial orbit in conjunction with ethmoid sinusitis. The abscess develops when infection breaks through the lamina papyracea or travels through the anterior or posterior ethmoidal foramina. The subperiosteal fluid collection can expand rapidly and may lead to blindness by compromising optic nerve function through several possible mechanisms: direct optic nerve compression, elevation of intraorbital pressure, or proptosis causing a stretch optic neuropathy [59]. Even with aggressive medical and surgical intervention, about 15% to 30% of patients who have SPA develop various visual sequelae [60].

Diagnosis. As in orbital cellulitis, ophthalmologic evaluation is essential. Clinically, SPA is suspected when a patient who has orbital cellulitis develops worsening proptosis and gaze restriction. The ability to distinguish colors may be used as a guide of disease progression because increasing intraorbital pressure causes loss of red/green perception before deterioration of visual acuity [51].

On CT images, axial views optimally demonstrate the displacement of the medial rectus muscle and the abscess within the orbit, whereas coronal cuts (Fig. 5) are useful to delineate orbital and sinus anatomy. With contrast-enhanced CT, the SPA is seen as a contrast-enhancing mass in the extraconal space. The ring-enhanced lesion or air-fluid level is pathognomonic for an SPA. Marked proptosis is seen, occasionally with a conic deformity of the posterior aspect of the globe. Osteomyelitis of the orbital wall can be seen in advanced cases. Extension of the inflammatory process into the intraconal space appears on CT as an ill-defined infiltration of the orbital fat with obliteration of optic nerve and extraocular muscles [54]. Depending on the size of the abscess, the adjacent rectus muscle is generally displaced inward and enlarged. One recent study used a lateral displacement of the medial rectus muscles of at least 2 mm as a diagnostic criterion for an SPA [61].

Treatment and choice of surgical approach. Controversy exists about the optimal initial management of SPA, especially in children. Although intravenous antibiotic therapy should be started immediately, some

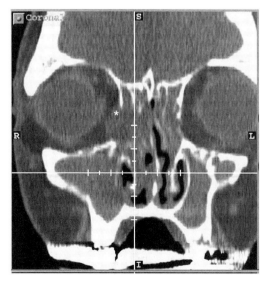

Fig. 5. Preoperative coronal CT without contrast demonstrating right inferomedial SPA from direct extension from right ethmoid sinusitis through the lamina papyracea (*asterisk*). (*Courtesy of* Rakesh Chandra, MD, Chicago, IL.)

otolaryngologists advocate immediate surgical drainage, whereas others recommend medical management, reserving surgery for nonresponders. Several
earlier studies concluded that the responsiveness of SPA to medical treatment appears to be age associated, with younger children thought to have
less virulent infections than older children [58,61–63]. Their inclusion criteria for medical management were age younger than 9 years, absence of frontal sinusitis, medial location of the abscess, absence of gas in the abscess
cavity, small abscess volume, nonrecurrent SPA, absence of acute optic
nerve or retinal compromise, and a nonodontogenic infection. Surgical
drainage was reserved for deterioration in visual acuity, appearance of an
afferent pupillary defect, continuing fever after 36 hours, clinical deterioration after 48 hours, or no improvement after 72 hours of medical treatment.
In a more recent study by Oxford and McClay [64], in contrast to prior
series, older children with SPA were managed successfully with medical
therapy. The ages of the 18 patients treated medically were not statistically
different from the 25 patients treated surgically. During hospitalization, the
most common antibiotics used were cefuroxime, clindamycin, vancomycin,
ceftriaxone, nafcillin, and gentamicin, with multiple antibiotics used in 65%
of the patients. Oxford proposed the following criteria for medical management of medial SPA:

- Normal vision, pupil, and retina
- No ophthalmoplegia
- Intraocular pressure of less than 20 mm Hg
- Proptosis of 5 mm or less
- Abscess width of 4 mm or less

Thus, it seems that a subset of patients who have SPA can be treated in this
manner with close ophthalmologic and otolaryngologic follow-up.

Surgical approaches to draining SPA include external, endoscopic, and
combined approaches. The traditional approach to medial SPA and orbital
abscess drainage has been by external ethmoidectomy, through a Lynch incision. In 1993, Manning [65] published the first case review that advocated
the endoscopic approach to treat SPA in children, which has since become
a widely accepted alternative to open approaches. The main limitation of the
endoscopic approach in this setting is the potential for increased bleeding of
the acutely inflamed mucosa [60,66].

The endoscopic technique involves ethmoidectomy, skeletonizing of the
lamina papyracea, and drainage of the orbital collection by cracking the
lamina with a Cottle or Freer elevator. Care should be taken not to violate
the periorbita. The intraoperative measurement of orbital pressures is
extremely helpful and often dictates the extent of orbital decompression.
In adults, postoperative care is performed as in routine sinus surgery. Patients are instructed to perform nasal saline irrigations, and endoscopic
debridements are performed in the office setting after 1 week. Although several studies [67,68] involving pediatric patients undergoing endoscopic sinus

surgery (ESS) found no effect on facial growth, conservative surgical resection in children undergoing ESS is generally advocated. Malik and colleagues [69] described a technique of immediate lamina papyracea reconstruction during endoscopic drainage of SPA to preserve as much facial skeleton as possible.

The transcaruncular approach in conjunction with endoscopic sinus drainage is an example of a combined approach that has been in use since 1996 by Pelton and colleagues [70]. It can replace external ethmoidectomy when the endoscopic attempt at draining the SPA has to be abandoned secondary to poor visualization from bleeding and inflammation. In the transcaruncular approach, an incision is made with tenotomy scissors between the caruncle and the semilunar fold. Dissection then proceeds posteriorly to the anterior medial orbital wall while protecting the globe and canalicular system. The orbital periosteum is incised sharply and elevated with a Freer until the abscess cavity is encountered. The transcaruncular approach to the medial orbital wall allows easy access and visualization of the abscess cavity from the orbital side of the lamina papyracea, without a cutaneous scar. Patient outcomes, in terms of length of stay and resolution of symptoms, were no different from those when treatment was endoscopic drainage alone. When used in conjunction with ESS, this technique allows confirmation of complete drainage on both the nasal and orbital sides.

Although less frequent, nonmedial SPAs can occur along the superior and inferior orbits, secondary to frontal sinusitis and maxillary sinusitis. SPAs located superiorly and laterally do not appear amenable to endoscopic drainage, and should be approached through external ethmoidectomy and lateral orbitotomy, respectively [66].

Orbital abscess

If orbital abscess is present as a sequela of paranasal sinusitis, progression to this stage can often be linked to a delay in diagnosis and therapy, or an immunocompromised state. Orbital abscesses may occur inside or outside the muscle cone when orbital cellulitis coalesces into a discrete collection of pus [54].

Diagnosis. Clinically, patients who have orbital abscesses have marked proptosis, chemosis, complete ophthalmoplegia, and visual impairment, with a risk for progression to irreversible blindness. Purulent material may drain spontaneously through the lid [60]. CT scanning will show diffuse infiltration of the intraconal and extraconal orbit fat, areas of cavitation that appear radiolucent. Associated radiographic findings are the presence of massive proptosis, extraocular enlargement, and, occasionally, gas formation. On MRI, a true necrotic abscess appears as an area of hypointensity on T1-weighted images and as an area of hyperintensity on T2-weighted images [54].

Treatment. When an abscess develops within the confines of the orbit, drainage is mandatory. Treatment consists of drainage of the involved sinuses and the abscess. Endoscopic drainage of medial orbital abscesses essentially involves the same technique as for SPA, with a few exceptions. Incision of the periorbita is usually necessary to drain an intraorbital abscess. A sickle knife can be used and the incision is made from posterior to anterior, thus affording good drainage of most extraconal abscesses. Posterior ethmoidectomy is indicated if there is significant posterior ethmoid disease and extension of the abscess toward the orbital apex. A wide exposure and decompression of the medial orbital wall may be necessary, especially if the orbital pressures continue to elevate substantially. Drainage of intraconal abscesses is best achieved through a combined approach and should never be attempted without participation of an ophthalmologist [60].

Cavernous sinus thrombosis

Cavernous sinus thrombosis (CST) results from the spread of infection from sinonasal cavities (sphenoid > ethmoid > frontal), or from infection of the middle third of the face. The syndrome can also occur as a complication of orbital cellulitis. The freely anastomosing, valveless venous system of the paranasal sinuses allows the spread of infection to the cavernous sinus in a retrograde fashion by way of the superior and inferior ophthalmic veins. Extension of phlebitis posteriorly into the cavernous sinus results in a progression of symptoms in the opposite eye, and serves as a distinguishing feature of CST. Although offending organisms may be aerobic or anaerobic, *S aureus* has been identified as the most common pathogen [54,71]. Even with rapid recognition and treatment, this condition may progress to loss of vision, meningitis, and even death.

Diagnosis. It is important, but difficult, to differentiate orbital cellulitis or abscess from a developing CST because of the life-threatening nature of the latter. The most important clinical signs include bilateral orbital involvement, rapidly progressive chemosis and ophthalmoplegia, severe retinal engorgement, fever to 105°F, and prostration. The most common signs of CST are related to the anatomic structures affected within the cavernous sinus, and result from direct injury to cranial nerves III through VI and impaired venous drainage from the orbit and the eye. Obstruction of venous drainage from the retina can result in papilledema, retinal hemorrhages, and visual loss. Spread to the contralateral cavernous sinus (by way of intercavernous sinuses) usually occurs within 24 to 48 hours of the initial presentation. Carotid thrombosis may follow CST with concomitant strokes, subdural empyema, brain abscess, or meningitis [71].

The diagnosis is best made on clinical grounds and confirmed by radiographic findings. Contrast-enhanced CT scans (Fig. 6) may reveal the source of infection, thickening of the superior ophthalmic vein, and irregular filling defects in the cavernous sinus. MRI using flow parameters and MR

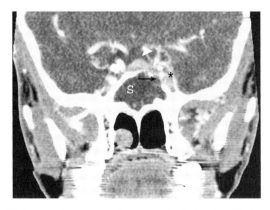

Fig. 6. Coronal CT sinuses with contrast demonstrating left sphenoid sinusitis (S) with bone erosion (*black arrow*). Note the filling defect and expansion of the left cavernous sinus consistent with CST (*asterisk*), and an abscess formed around the supraclinoid internal carotid artery (*arrowhead*). (*Courtesy of* Ilana Seligman, MD, Chicago, IL.)

venogram is a more sensitive method than CT for diagnosing CST. MR reveals engorgement of the cavernous sinus, ophthalmic veins, and extraocular muscles. The cavernous portion of the internal carotid artery is usually deformed. The signal from the abnormal cavernous sinus is heterogeneous, and an obvious hyperintense signal of thrombosed vascular sinuses may be seen on all pulse sequences. Mycotic (septic) aneurysm of the internal carotid artery is a serious complication of CST; it can be suspected on CT and MRI scans and confirmed by standard angiography [54].

Treatment. Treatment includes high-dose intravenous antibiotics that cross the blood–brain barrier and are directed at the most common pathogens associated with the disease. Empiric treatment may include nafcillin, ceftriaxone, metronidazole, or vancomycin if methicillin-resistant *S aureus* is a concern. Patients who have CST are usually treated with intravenous antibiotics for 3 to 4 weeks, or for 6 to 8 weeks if intracranial complication is evident. Surgical intervention, consisting of drainage of the affected sinuses, is advisable in most circumstances. Close observation for signs of continued sepsis, extension of septic thrombus, or metastatic infection is necessary. The role of anticoagulation to minimize the progression of thrombosis is contentious because its efficacy is undetermined, and prospective trials of anticoagulation may never be performed because of the rarity of this condition. Nevertheless, retrospective reviews of published reports indicate that hemorrhage caused by anticoagulation is rare, and that early adjunctive anticoagulation is beneficial in these patients if commenced after excluding the hemorrhagic sequelae of CST radiologically [72]. One study suggested that heparin use in conjunction with antibiotics early in the course of CST may reduce morbidity, but found no conclusive evidence that it reduces mortality [73]. Steroid therapy is not recommended [71].

Intracranial complications

Intracranial complications of sinusitis (ICS) are uncommon but potentially devastating. For patients hospitalized with rhinosinusitis, the incidence of intracranial extension ranges from 3.7% to 11% [19,74]. ICS include meningitis, epidural abscess, subdural abscess, intracerebral abscess, and venous sinus thrombosis, as shown in Table 2. In the largest series to date, consisting of 219 pediatric and adult patients, Singh and colleagues [75] found subdural abscess (58%) to be the most common ICS. Published series continue to differ widely on the relative frequencies of each of these complications.

The ability of bacterial infection to extend intracranially is related to the location of the paranasal sinuses and the unique venous relationship of this area. The pathogenesis of ICS includes two major mechanisms: direct extension and retrograde thrombophlebitis by way of the valveless diploe veins. The frontal sinus forms within calvarial bone that contains diploe. Draining the diploe is a complicated anastomosis of valveless veins that communicate with the venous plexus of the dura, scalp, and periorbita [76]. It has been suggested that adolescents and young adults are most affected because it is at this age that the valveless diploic system is at its most vascular [77,78].

Table 2
Intracranial complications of sinusitis

	Sinus source	Clinical presentation
Meningitis	Sphenoid, ethmoid	Acute and rapidly progressive; fever, headache, changes in mental status, photophobia, and meningismus
Epidural abscess	Frontal	Slowly expanding, indolent onset; headache, fever, and local pain and tenderness
Subdural abscess	Frontal	Rapidly progressive, neurosurgical emergency; headache, fever, lethargy, meningeal signs, seizures
Intracerebral abscess	Frontal	Asymptomatic phase, followed by headache, fever, vomiting, and lethargy; frontal lobe abscess; mood and behavioral changes
Cavernous sinus thrombosis	Sphenoid, ethmoid	Proptosis, ophthalmoplegia, chemosis, decreased visual acuity, V1 and V2 facial anesthesia; involvement of the contralateral eye is a late finding
Superior sagittal sinus thrombosis	Frontal	Patients are extremely ill, with high spiking fevers, meningeal signs, and neurologic defects

(*Data from* Giannoni CM, Weinberger DG. Complications of rhinosinusitis. In: Bailey BJ, Johnson JT, Newlands SD, et al, editors. Head & neck surgery – otolaryngology. Vol. 1. 4th edition. Philadelphia: Lippincott Williams & Wilkins; 2006. p. 494–504.)

In adults, ICS were more commonly seen in patients who had a history of chronic rhinosinusitis [38,76]. In the pediatric population, ICS were essentially caused exclusively by acute sinusitis, with no patient having a significant history or symptoms of chronic sinus disease [78–81]. Anaerobes (*Streptococcus, Bacteroides*), *S aureus*, other *Streptococcus* sp, and *H influenzae* are the most commonly isolated organisms in children and adults with ICS [38].

Several series [78,81,82] found that extracranial complications, especially orbital infections, not only commonly coexisted with ICS but also dominated the presentation of most of the children whose intracranial infections were otherwise silent. A retrospective chart review by Herrmann and Forsen [82] identified risk factors for intracranial extension in children admitted for orbital complications of acute rhinosinusitis. These risk factors included age 7 years and older, failure to improve after appropriate therapy, changes in neurologic status, frontal sinus opacification on CT, superior or lateral position of orbital abscess, need for surgical intervention to drain orbital abscess, male sex, and African-American race. When evaluating a child presenting with orbital or forehead swelling and sinusitis, it is important to consider the possibility of a concurrent intracranial infection, even in the absence of neurologic findings.

The overall mortality rate of ICS has been declining, to approximately 4% in recent series [76,78,80,81]. In contrast, these series report significant rates of morbidity (13%–35%), including long-term neurologic deficits, cognitive impairment, cranial nerve palsy, aphasia, epilepsy, hydrocephalus, and visual and hearing loss.

Meningitis

The source of meningitis is usually the sphenoid or ethmoid sinuses. In a review of 21 patients who had meningitis secondary to sinusitis, Younis [83] reported that all adult patients had evidence of sphenoid sinusitis on CT. Neurologic sequelae are common in patients who have meningitis, primarily seizure disorders and sensorineural deficits, including a 25% incidence of hearing loss [19]. The most common organism is *Streptococcus pneumoniae* [25,38].

Diagnosis. Symptoms include high fever, changes in mental status, photophobia, meningismus, and severe headache, superimposed on the rhinosinusitis complaints. Patients may be toxic and may demonstrate cranial nerve palsies. They may also display behavior changes, vomiting, and seizures. Although CT remains the standard initial modality for diagnosis of sinusitis or sinusitis with complications, MRI is mandatory when intracranial extension is suspected. For patients who have meningitis, the CT scan of the brain is usually normal. However, contrast-enhanced MRI typically shows dural enhancement, usually most evident along the falx cerebri, tentorium, and convexity dura [84]. If imaging studies show no evidence of increased intracranial pressure, a lumbar puncture should be done for cytologic and laboratory analysis of the sample; however, it may be unnecessary in those with proven focal intracranial suppuration on scanning, and may be potentially dangerous because of the risk of uncal herniation [76].

Treatment. The initial and mainstay treatment of meningitis is administration of broad-spectrum intravenous antibiotics that cross the blood–brain barrier. Most institutions recommend a third generation parenteral cephalosporin and metronidazole for empiric therapy. Although intravenous steroids have been shown to reduce the incidence of hearing loss from meningitis originating from otitis media, the benefits of steroid use in meningitis of sinogenic origin remain unproved and controversial [25]. Consensus does not exist at this time on the role and timing of endoscopic sinus surgery in the treatment of meningitis, secondary to lack of randomized controlled studies comparing outcomes of medical to combined medical and surgical treatments. Most institutions recommend surgical drainage of the sinuses if clinical improvement is not evident 24 to 48 hours after the start of intravenous antibiotics, provided the patient has been stabilized [19,25,38,83,85]. Others believe that the early use of functional endoscopic surgery in patients who have ICS has the potential to accelerate clinical improvement considerably, recommending surgery as part of their routine management [77,81]. The overall mortality rate reported for community-acquired meningitis is 25% and that for nosocomial meningitis is 35% [86].

Epidural abscess

Epidural abscess was found to be the most common intracranial complication of sinusitis in three large pediatric series [53,81,87]. Epidural abscesses form between the skull and dura and expand slowly because of the tight adherence of dura to bone. This type of infection is seen almost exclusively in patients who have frontal sinusitis, probably secondary to the high degree of venous communication and loosely adherent dura in that particular site. Patients may have a prolonged period, up to several weeks, of nonspecific symptoms until either the infection penetrates the dura or the abscess becomes large enough to cause elevated intracranial pressure [81].

Diagnosis. Symptoms are commonly mild and may include fever, headache, and scalp pain and swelling, evolving over several weeks. Frank neurologic deficits are usually absent and diagnosis is made using contrasted CT or MRI (Fig. 7). The most common organisms are *S aureus* and *Streptococci* [19].

Treatment. Epidural abscesses have a favorable prognosis regardless of the origin of infection, but, unlike meningitis, they usually require both medical and surgical treatment. High-dose broad-spectrum intravenous antibiotics

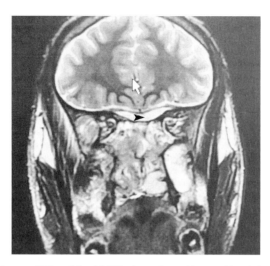

Fig. 7. Enhanced coronal T2-weighted MRI of a patient with an epidural abscess (*black arrowhead*) above the planum sphenoidale. (*Courtesy of* Rakesh Chandra, MD, Chicago, IL.)

should be started immediately and surgical management requires coordination between otolaryngology and neurosurgery services, most commonly concurrent drainage of the sinuses and epidural abscess. Sinuses can be addressed through ESS, frontal sinus trephination, or combined approaches. The epidural abscess is most commonly addressed through craniotomy. Other approaches include burr holes, or through paranasal sinuses if a solitary epidural abscess is observed adjacent to bony dehiscence in the skull base [81,87,88]. In rare cases, cranialization of the frontal sinus may be necessary if inspection of the posterior table reveals marked osteitis with perforation or necrosis [81].

Although the standard management of epidural abscess involves drainage, one series by Heran and colleagues [88] describes effective treatment without an intracranial procedure; a small group of patients were treated with only sinus drainage and antibiotics for at least 6 weeks. Abscesses had a mean size of 3 × 3 × 1 cm (length, width, depth) and CT follow-up revealed minimal or no enlargement of the abscess or mass effect at 1 week, a decrease or stable size at 2 weeks, and resolution by 6 weeks. It was concluded that such conservative management can be applied to patients presenting without focal neurologic deficits or increased intracranial pressure, and with no intradural infection. Future studies with larger numbers of patients are needed to validate these findings, compare the outcomes with standard therapy, and formulate an algorithmic approach.

Subdural abscess

A subdural abscess is usually precipitated by a frontal or ethmoid sinus infection, and, because of the lack of boundaries, subdural empyema commonly spreads diffusely within the subdural space (ie, over the cerebral convexities, in the interhemispheric fissure and along the tentorium, in the posterior fossa, and, in some cases, into the spinal canal) [19,88]. Mortality has been reported to be as high as 25%, with an additional morbidity in approximately 30% of the survivors [19].

Diagnosis. The presenting symptoms of subdural abscess are reflective of increased intracranial pressure, meningeal irritation, and cerebritis. The most common symptoms include headache, fever, and neck stiffness. With rapid progression, patients can display a depressed level of consciousness, focal neurologic deficits or cranial nerve palsies, hemiparesis, papilledema, vomiting, and septic shock. Seizures occur in 25% to 80% of cases and are more common with subdural abscesses than with other ICS [19,89].

CT is helpful in making the diagnosis; however, it may not show a fluid collection in early cases. When visualized on CT, subdural abscess appears as a thin, hypodense subdural lesion, with linear enhancement of the medial surface. Mass effect is usually caused by ischemia and edema rather than from the abscess. MRI with gadolinium enhancement allows better evaluation of the brain [89]. Infections are usually polymicrobial, and the collection can have multiple loculations. Lumbar puncture is contraindicated in patients who have subdural abscess secondary to possible increased intracranial pressure. Neurologic deterioration and transtentorial herniation after lumbar puncture are well described and have led to death [78].

Treatment. Broad-spectrum intravenous antibiotics and surgical drainage of the underlying sinusitis and subdural abscess constitute treatment options. Recommended empiric therapy is a third-generation cephalosporin plus metronidazole for good cerebrospinal fluid and abscess penetration. The length of antibiotic therapy is variable and can range from 2 weeks to 6 to 8 weeks if osteomyelitis is evident. Drainage of the subdural abscess can be accomplished through craniotomy or burr holes; controversy exists in the neurosurgical literature regarding the preferred intervention. Some patients treated with burr holes require additional surgery or conversion to craniotomy; however, both procedures are considered acceptable [19,25,89]. Additional care includes prophylactic anticonvulsants. Corticosteroids have been advocated by some for use in patients who have an acute clinical deterioration or significant cerebral edema but others argue against their use secondary to interference with antibiotic penetration and host immunologic response [25].

Intracerebral abscess

The most common locations for intracerebral abscess are the frontal and frontoparietal lobes, respectively. Frontal sinusitis is usually the precipitating site, although involvement of the ethmoid and sphenoid sinuses has also been reported [19]. Temporal lobe abscesses are uncommonly associated with paranasal sinusitis, although sphenoid sinusitis may be the culprit [38]. Thrombophlebitis and septic implantation in areas of sluggish venous flow seem to be the predominant routes of parenchymal abscess formation, with the junction of white and gray matter at highest risk. Brain abscesses are associated with high mortality, as high as 20% to 30%, with approximately 60% of children who survive developing neurologic and developmental sequelae [19].

Diagnosis. A cerebral abscess begins as an area of cerebritis, with associated headache. A quiescent, asymptomatic phase follows while the abscess coalesces. Abscesses localized to the frontal lobe are associated with more subtle symptoms, such as mood and behavioral changes. Headache and lethargy may be experienced as the abscess expands. Seizures and focal neurologic deficits can occur, and the presence of these signs is associated with increased long-term morbidity and mortality [74]. Abscess rupture can occur and is often fatal. Imaging is diagnostic and MRI demonstrates a cystic lesion with a distinct hypointense strongly enhancing capsule on T2-weighted images. Lumbar puncture can be life threatening and its risks outweigh any diagnostic benefit.

Treatment. Neurosurgical consultation should be obtained early and a treatment plan should be initiated. Treatment involves broad-spectrum intravenous antibiotics with good cerebrospinal fluid penetration, and surgical drainage of the affected sinuses. The effective treatment of intracerebral abscess remains controversial; it depends on the patient's condition, the maturity of the abscess wall, and the location of the abscess in the brain. Some may resolve with medical therapy, whereas others have to be treated surgically. Surgical options include stereotactic aspiration and drainage versus open surgical excision [90].

Venous sinus thrombosis (superior sagittal and cavernous sinuses)
   Infection spreads to the cavernous and sagittal sinuses by way of retrograde thrombophlebitis secondary to frontal sinusitis. CST was discussed earlier under orbital complications. Sagittal sinus thrombosis is usually found in association with other complications such as subdural, epidural, or intracerebral abscesses [25,38,76].

Diagnosis. Clinical severity depends on the extent of the thrombosis and the vessels involved. Acute occlusion of the dural sinus is usually not well tolerated and may lead to massive cerebral edema, venous congestion, and infarction. Patients are extremely ill, presenting with high spiking fevers, meningeal signs, or other serious neurologic complications. Occasionally, patients who have dural sinus thrombosis present with mild symptoms because of an incomplete occlusion or because of well-established collaterals [85]. MRI may reveal focal defects of enhancement after gadolinium administration, and MR angiogram and venogram can further delineate the process.

Treatment. Treatment includes high-dose intravenous antibiotics and drainage of the involved paranasal sinuses. Systemic anticoagulant therapy is used, and is continued until radiologic evidence of resolution of the thrombus is obtained; however, results have been inconsistent [76,85]. The treatment of choice for acute major dural sinus thrombosis is still controversial. Surgical reconstruction of a thrombosed sinus has been described but has not gained widespread acceptance. Reports [91] have demonstrated the benefits of open surgical thrombectomy combined with direct endovascular thrombolysis therapy, specifically urokinase or streptokinase infused into the superior sagittal sinus by a catheter placed through a burr-hole craniotomy. Illustrating recent improvements in interventional techniques and catheter technology, two studies [85,92] described successful direct thrombolysis in acute dural sinus thrombosis by way of selective venography through a femoral vein.

References

[1] deShazo RD, O'Brien M, Chapin K, et al. A new classification and diagnostic criteria for invasive fungal sinusitis. Arch Otolaryngol Head Neck Surg 1997;123(11):1181–8.

[2] deShazo RD. Fungal sinusitis. Am J Med Sci 1998;316(1):39–45.

[3] Stringer SP, Ryan MW. Chronic invasive fungal rhinosinusitis. Otolaryngol Clin North Am 2000;33(2):375–87.

[4] Ferguson BJ. Definitions of fungal rhinosinusitis. Otolaryngol Clin North Am 2000;33(2): 227–35.

[5] Gillespie MB, O'Malley BW. An algorithmic approach to the diagnosis and management of invasive fungal rhinosinusitis in the immunocompromised patient. Otolaryngol Clin North Am 2000;33(2):323–34.

[6] Chopra H, Dua K, Malhotra V, et al. Invasive fungal sinusitis of isolated sphenoid sinus in immunocompetent subjects. Mycoses 2006;49(1):30–6.

[7] Sridhara SR, Paragache G, Panda NK, et al. Mucormycosis in immunocompetent individuals: an increasing trend. J Otolaryngol 2005;34(6):402–6.

[8] Park AH, Muntz HR, Smith ME, et al. Pediatric invasive fungal rhinosinusitis in immunocompromised children with cancer. Otolaryngol Head Neck Surg 2005;133(3):411–6.

[9] Gillespie MB, O'Malley BW Jr, Francis HW. An approach to fulminant invasive fungal rhinosinusitis in the immunocompromised host. Arch Otolaryngol Head Neck Surg 1998; 124(5):520–6.

[10] DelGaudio JM, Swain RE Jr, Kingdom TT, et al. Computed tomographic findings in patients with invasive fungal sinusitis. Arch Otolaryngol Head Neck Surg 2003;129(2): 236–40.

[11] Silverman CS, Mancuso AA. Periantral soft-tissue infiltration and its relevance to the early detection of invasive fungal sinusitis: CT and MR findings. AJNR Am J Neuroradiol 1998; 19(2):321–5.

[12] Schell WA. Histopathology of fungal rhinosinusitis. Otolaryngol Clin North Am 2000;33(2): 251–76.

[13] Sahin B, Paydas S, Cosar E, et al. Role of granulocyte colony-stimulating factor in the treatment of mucormycosis. Eur J Clin Microbiol Infect Dis 1996;15(11):866–9.

[14] Parikh SL, Venkatraman G, DelGaudio JM. Invasive fungal sinusitis: a 15-year review from a single institution. Am J Rhinol 2004;18(2):75–81.

[15] Herbrecht R, Denning DW, Patterson TF, et al. Voriconazole versus amphotericin B for primary therapy of invasive aspergillosis. N Engl J Med 2002;347(6):408–15.

[16] Kennedy CA, Adams GL, Neglia JP, et al. Impact of surgical treatment on paranasal fungal infections in bone marrow transplant patients. Otolaryngol Head Neck Surg 1997;116 (6 Pt 1):610–6.

[17] Denning DW. Therapeutic outcome in invasive aspergillosis. Clin Infect Dis 1996;23(3): 608–15.

[18] Ferguson BJ. Mucormycosis of the nose and paranasal sinuses. Otolaryngol Clin North Am 2000;33(2):349–65.

[19] Younis RT, Lazar RH, Anand VK. Intracranial complications of sinusitis: a 15-year review of 39 cases. Ear Nose Throat J 2002;81(9):636–8, 640–32, 644.

[20] Jackson LL, Kountakis SE. Classification and management of rhinosinusitis and its complications. Otolaryngol Clin North Am 2005;38(6):1143–53.

[21] Arrue P, Kany MT, Serrano E, et al. Mucoceles of the paranasal sinuses: uncommon location. J Laryngol Otol 1998;112(9):840–4.

[22] Eggesbo HB. Radiological imaging of inflammatory lesions in the nasal cavity and paranasal sinuses. Eur Radiol 2006;16(4):872–88.

[23] Kosling S, Hintner M, Brandt S, et al. Mucoceles of the sphenoid sinus. Eur J Radiol 2004; 51(1):1–5.

[24] Haloi AK, Ditchfield M, Maixner W. Mucocele of the sphenoid sinus. Pediatr Radiol 2006; 36(9):987–90.

[25] Goldberg AN, Oroszlan G, Anderson TD. Complications of frontal sinusitis and their management. Otolaryngol Clin North Am 2001;34(1):211–25.

[26] Har-El G. Transnasal endoscopic management of frontal mucoceles. Otolaryngol Clin North Am 2001;34(1):243–51.

[27] Lanzieri CF, Shah M, Krauss D, et al. Use of gadolinium-enhanced MR imaging for differentiating mucoceles from neoplasms in the paranasal sinuses. Radiology 1991;178(2): 425–8.

[28] Har-El G, DiMaio T. Histologic and physiologic studies of marsupialized sinus mucoceles: report of two cases. J Otolaryngol 2000;29(4):195–8.

[29] Lund VJ, Milroy CM. Fronto-ethmoidal mucocoeles: a histopathological analysis. J Laryngol Otol 1991;105(11):921–3.

[30] Lund VJ. Endoscopic management of paranasal sinus mucocoeles. J Laryngol Otol 1998; 112(1):36–40.

[31] Kennedy DW, Josephson JS, Zinreich SJ, et al. Endoscopic sinus surgery for mucoceles: a viable alternative. Laryngoscope 1989;99(9):885–95.

[32] Har-El G. Endoscopic management of 108 sinus mucoceles. Laryngoscope 2001;111(12): 2131–4.

[33] Khong JJ, Malhotra R, Selva D, et al. Efficacy of endoscopic sinus surgery for paranasal sinus mucocele including modified endoscopic Lothrop procedure for frontal sinus mucocele. J Laryngol Otol 2004;118(5):352–6.

[34] Weber AL. Inflammatory diseases of the paranasal sinuses and mucoceles. Otolaryngol Clin North Am 1988;21(3):421–37.

[35] Flamm ES. Percivall Pott: an 18th century neurosurgeon. J Neurosurg 1992;76(2):319–26.

[36] Kombogiorgas D, Solanki GA. The Pott puffy tumor revisited: neurosurgical implications of this unforgotten entity. Case report and review of the literature. J Neurosurg 2006; 105(Suppl 2):143–9.

[37] Bambakidis NC, Cohen AR. Intracranial complications of frontal sinusitis in children: Pott's puffy tumor revisited. Pediatr Neurosurg 2001;35(2):82–9.

[38] Giannoni CM, Stewart MG, Alford EL. Intracranial complications of sinusitis. Laryngoscope 1997;107(7):863–7.

[39] Thomas JN, Nel JR. Acute spreading osteomyelitis of the skull complicating frontal sinusitis. J Laryngol Otol 1977;91(1):55–62.

[40] Bordley JE, Bischofberger W. Osteomyelitis of the frontal bone. Laryngoscope 1967;77(8): 1234–44.

[41] Feder HM Jr, Cates KL, Cementina AM. Pott puffy tumor: a serious occult infection. Pediatrics 1987;79(4):625–9.

[42] Verbon A, Husni RN, Gordon SM, et al. Pott's puffy tumor due to Haemophilus influenzae: case report and review. Clin Infect Dis 1996;23(6):1305–7.

[43] Guillen A, Brell M, Cardona E, et al. Pott's puffy tumour: still not an eradicated entity. Childs Nerv Syst 2001;17(6):359–62.

[44] Wells RG, Sty JR, Landers AD. Radiological evaluation of Pott puffy tumor. JAMA 1986; 255(10):1331–3.

[45] Turner WJ, Davidson TM. Endoscopic management of acute frontal sinusitis. Ear Nose Throat J 1994;73(8):594–7.

[46] Elverland HH, Melheim I, Anke IM. Acute orbit from ethmoiditis drained by endoscopic sinus surgery. Acta Otolaryngol Suppl 1992;492:147–51.

[47] Quraishi H, Zevallos JP. Subdural empyema as a complication of sinusitis in the pediatric population. Int J Pediatr Otorhinolaryngol 2006;70(9):1581–6.

[48] van der Merwe J. Functional endoscopic sinus surgery–the South African experience. S Afr J Surg 1994;32(2):67–9.

[49] Mortimore S, Wormald PJ. Management of acute complicated sinusitis: a 5-year review. Otolaryngol Head Neck Surg 1999;121(5):639–42.

[50] Williamson-Noble FA. Diseases of the orbit and its contents, secondary to pathological conditions of the nose and paranasal sinuses. Ann R Coll Surg Engl 1954;15(1):46–64.

[51] Osguthorpe JD, Hochman M. Inflammatory sinus diseases affecting the orbit. Otolaryngol Clin North Am 1993;26(4):657–71.

[52] Chandler JR, Langenbrunner DJ, Stevens ER. The pathogenesis of orbital complications in acute sinusitis. Laryngoscope 1970;80(9):1414–28.

[53] Oxford LE, McClay J. Complications of acute sinusitis in children. Otolaryngol Head Neck Surg 2005;133(1):32–7.

[54] Eustis HS, Mafee MF, Walton C, et al. MR imaging and CT of orbital infections and complications in acute rhinosinusitis. Radiol Clin North Am 1998;36(6):1165–83, xi.

[55] Younis RT, Lazar RH, Bustillo A, et al. Orbital infection as a complication of sinusitis: are diagnostic and treatment trends changing? Ear Nose Throat J 2002;81(11):771–5.

[56] Donahue SP, Schwartz G. Preseptal and orbital cellulitis in childhood. A changing microbiologic spectrum. Ophthalmology 1998;105(10):1902–5 [discussion: 1905–6].

[57] Jackson K, Baker SR. Clinical implications of orbital cellulitis. Laryngoscope 1986;96(5): 568–74.

[58] Harris GJ. Subperiosteal abscess of the orbit. Age as a factor in the bacteriology and response to treatment. Ophthalmology 1994;101(3):585–95.

[59] Harris GJ. Subperiosteal abscess of the orbit. Arch Ophthalmol 1983;101(5):751–7.

[60] Fakhri S, Pereira K. Endoscopic management of orbital abscesses. Otolaryngol Clin North Am 2006;39(5):1037–47, viii.

[61] Brown CL, Graham SM, Griffin MC, et al. Pediatric medial subperiosteal orbital abscess: medical management where possible. Am J Rhinol 2004;18(5):321–7.

[62] Garcia GH, Harris GJ. Criteria for nonsurgical management of subperiosteal abscess of the orbit: analysis of outcomes 1988–1998. Ophthalmology 2000;107(8):1454–6 [discussion: 1457–8].

[63] Harris GJ. Subperiosteal abscess of the orbit: older children and adults require aggressive treatment. Ophthal Plast Reconstr Surg 2001;17(6):395–7.

[64] Oxford LE, McClay J. Medical and surgical management of subperiosteal orbital abscess secondary to acute sinusitis in children. Int J Pediatr Otorhinolaryngol 2006;70(11): 1853–61.

[65] Manning SC. Endoscopic management of medial subperiosteal orbital abscess. Arch Otolaryngol Head Neck Surg 1993;119(7):789–91.
[66] Noordzij JP, Harrison SE, Mason JC, et al. Pitfalls in the endoscopic drainage of subperiosteal orbital abscesses secondary to sinusitis. Am J Rhinol 2002;16(2):97–101.
[67] Bothwell MR, Piccirillo JF, Lusk RP, et al. Long-term outcome of facial growth after functional endoscopic sinus surgery. Otolaryngol Head Neck Surg 2002;126(6):628–34.
[68] Senior B, Wirtschafter A, Mai C, et al. Quantitative impact of pediatric sinus surgery on facial growth. Laryngoscope 2000;110(11):1866–70.
[69] Malik V, Khwaja S, De Carpentier J. Immediate lamina papyracea reconstruction during endoscopic sinus surgery for surgically managed subperiosteal abscess in children. Laryngoscope 2006;116(5):835–8.
[70] Pelton RW, Smith ME, Patel BC, et al. Cosmetic considerations in surgery for orbital subperiosteal abscess in children: experience with a combined transcaruncular and transnasal endoscopic approach. Arch Otolaryngol Head Neck Surg 2003;129(6):652–5.
[71] Cannon ML, Antonio BL, McCloskey JJ, et al. Cavernous sinus thrombosis complicating sinusitis. Pediatr Crit Care Med 2004;5(1):86–8.
[72] Bhatia K, Jones NS. Septic cavernous sinus thrombosis secondary to sinusitis: are anticoagulants indicated? A review of the literature. J Laryngol Otol 2002;116(9):667–76.
[73] Levine SR, Twyman RE, Gilman S. The role of anticoagulation in cavernous sinus thrombosis. Neurology 1988;38(4):517–22.
[74] Clayman GL, Adams GL, Paugh DR, et al. Intracranial complications of paranasal sinusitis: a combined institutional review. Laryngoscope 1991;101(3):234–9.
[75] Singh B, Van Dellen J, Ramjettan S, et al. Sinogenic intracranial complications. J Laryngol Otol 1995;109(10):945–50.
[76] Gallagher RM, Gross CW, Phillips CD. Suppurative intracranial complications of sinusitis. Laryngoscope 1998;108(11 Pt 1):1635–42.
[77] Herrmann BW, Chung JC, Eisenbeis JF, et al. Intracranial complications of pediatric frontal rhinosinusitis. Am J Rhinol 2006;20(3):320–4.
[78] Jones NS, Walker JL, Bassi S, et al. The intracranial complications of rhinosinusitis: can they be prevented? Laryngoscope 2002;112(1):59–63.
[79] Lerner DN, Choi SS, Zalzal GH, et al. Intracranial complications of sinusitis in childhood. Ann Otol Rhinol Laryngol 1995;104(4 Pt 1):288–93.
[80] Giannoni C, Sulek M, Friedman EM. Intracranial complications of sinusitis: a pediatric series. Am J Rhinol 1998;12(3):173–8.
[81] Germiller JA, Monin DL, Sparano AM, et al. Intracranial complications of sinusitis in children and adolescents and their outcomes. Arch Otolaryngol Head Neck Surg 2006;132(9):969–76.
[82] Herrmann BW, Forsen JW Jr. Simultaneous intracranial and orbital complications of acute rhinosinusitis in children. Int J Pediatr Otorhinolaryngol 2004;68(5):619–25.
[83] Younis RT, Anand VK, Childress C. Sinusitis complicated by meningitis: current management. Laryngoscope 2001;111(8):1338–42.
[84] Younis RT, Anand VK, Davidson B. The role of computed tomography and magnetic resonance imaging in patients with sinusitis with complications. Laryngoscope 2002;112(2):224–9.
[85] Niwa J, Ohyama H, Matumura S, et al. Treatment of acute superior sagittal sinus thrombosis by t-PA infusion via venography–direct thrombolytic therapy in the acute phase. Surg Neurol 1998;49(4):425–9.
[86] Durand ML, Calderwood SB, Weber DJ, et al. Acute bacterial meningitis in adults. A review of 493 episodes. N Engl J Med 1993;328(1):21–8.
[87] Glickstein JS, Chandra RK, Thompson JW. Intracranial complications of pediatric sinusitis. Otolaryngol Head Neck Surg 2006;134(5):733–6.
[88] Heran NS, Steinbok P, Cochrane DD. Conservative neurosurgical management of intracranial epidural abscesses in children. Neurosurgery 2003;53(4):893–7 [discussion: 897–8].

[89] Osborn MK, Steinberg JP. Subdural empyema and other suppurative complications of paranasal sinusitis. Lancet Infect Dis 2007;7(1):62–7.

[90] Boviatsis EJ, Kouyialis AT, Stranjalis G, et al. CT-guided stereotactic aspiration of brain abscesses. Neurosurg Rev 2003;26(3):206–9.

[91] Higashida RT, Helmer E, Halbach VV, et al. Direct thrombolytic therapy for superior sagittal sinus thrombosis. AJNR Am J Neuroradiol 1989;10(Suppl 5):S4–6.

[92] Philips MF, Bagley LJ, Sinson GP, et al. Endovascular thrombolysis for symptomatic cerebral venous thrombosis. J Neurosurg 1999;90(1):65–71.

ELSEVIER
SAUNDERS

Otolaryngol Clin N Am
41 (2008) 525–536

OTOLARYNGOLOGIC
CLINICS
OF NORTH AMERICA

Epistaxis

Thomas O. Gifford, MD, Capt, MC, USAF[a], Richard R. Orlandi, MD, FACS[a,b,c,*,1]

[a]*Division of Otolaryngology – Head and Neck Surgery,
University of Utah School of Medicine, 50 North Medical Drive,
3C120, Salt Lake City, UT 84132, USA*
[b]*Center for Therapeutic Biomaterials, University of Utah School of Medicine,
50 North Medical Drive, 3C120, Salt Lake City, UT 84132, USA*
[c]*George E. Wahlen Veterans Affairs Medical Center,
50 North Medical Drive, 3C120, Salt Lake City, UT 84132, USA*

Epistaxis is a common occurrence. The estimated lifetime incidence of epistaxis is approximately 60% [1]. However, most episodes are minor in nature and do not require intervention or medical evaluation. Minor bleeding episodes occur more frequently in children and adolescents, whereas severe bleeds requiring otolaryngologic intervention often occur in individuals older than 50 [2]. The objective of this article is to review the common causes and treatment options for severe epistaxis, including surgical intervention.

Vascular anatomy

It is important to understand the vascular anatomy to apply the appropriate treatment modalities. Blood supply to the nasal cavity originates from both the internal and external carotid systems and contains multiple anastomoses, the most prominent of which is Kiesselbach's plexus in the anterior nasal septum.

The external carotid supplies the facial artery and internal maxillary artery (IMA). The superior labial artery derives from the facial artery and gives off branches near the columella that supply the anterior nasal septum.

The views expressed in this article are those of the authors and do not reflect the official policy or position of the United States Air Force, the Department of Defense, or the US Government.

[1] Dr. Orlandi is a consultant to, and a stockholder in, Carbylan BioSurgery, Inc., and a consultant to Medtronic ENT.

* Corresponding author.
E-mail address: richard.orlandi@hsc.utah.edu (R.R. Orlandi).

0030-6665/08/$ - see front matter. Published by Elsevier Inc.
doi:10.1016/j.otc.2008.01.003

The IMA courses through the pterygopalatine fossa and divides into multiple branches, terminating in the sphenopalatine artery (SPA), which enters the nasal cavity through the sphenopalatine foramen on the lateral nasal wall. The SPA typically divides into two branches upon passing through the foramen, but may divide into three or more branches. It may also divide within the pterygopalatine fossa, before passing through the foramen. These anomalies are of great importance during ligation of the artery because the surgeon must search for multiple vessels to treat bleeding from the SPA effectively. The two most common branches of the SPA are the nasopalatine artery, which supplies the posterior nasal septum, and a posterior superior branch, contributing to the middle and inferior turbinates. The descending palatine artery is the other terminal branch of the IMA, separating from the SPA within the medial portion of the pterygopalatine fossa. It traverses inferiorly within the greater palatine canal, travels anteriorly along the palate, and supplies the anterior septum through the incisive foramen.

The internal carotid artery system supplies the nasal cavity through the anterior and posterior ethmoidal arteries. These are branches of the ophthalmic artery, which enters the orbit with the optic nerve. These arteries enter the nasal cavity through foramina in the medial orbital wall, within the frontoethmoidal suture. The anterior ethmoidal foramen is located 24 mm posterior to the lacrimal crest. The posterior ethmoidal foramen can be found 12 mm posterior to the anterior one, although the posterior ethmoidal artery can be absent in up to one third of individuals [2]. The optic nerve is located 6 mm posterior to the posterior ethmoidal artery, when the artery is present. During open ligation of the ethmoidal arteries, these measurements serve as useful guides to prevent injury to the optic nerve. Once the ethmoidal arteries leave the orbit, they course medially along the roof of the ethmoid sinuses and supply the nasal septum. The anterior ethmoid artery crosses the roof of the ethmoid sinuses just posterior to the frontal sinus ostium. The artery's position may be within the ethmoid roof or, occasionally, may lie more inferiorly, within a bony partition that acts like a mesentery. In this situation, it is more easily injured during endoscopic procedures (Fig. 1) [3].

Causes of epistaxis

Epistaxis results from a multitude of causes, both local and systemic [2,4,5]. Common local factors include digital trauma, nasal septal deviation, neoplasia, and chemical irritants, whereas coagulopathies, renal failure, alcoholism, and vascular abnormalities are common systemic factors. A personal or family history of frequent bleeding, heavy bleeding, or easy bruising suggests a systemic bleeding disorder. Although these conditions are rarely the cause of epistaxis, a thorough investigation is indicated in these patients to rule out systemic disease. Likewise, epistaxis is rarely caused by neoplasm, but persistent unilateral bleeding should prompt a nasal endoscopy and possibly radiologic imaging to rule out a tumor.

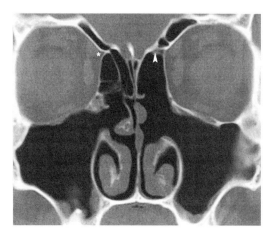

Fig. 1. Anterior ethmoid arteries. The left artery (*arrowhead*) crosses the skull base in a bone partition, leaving an air space posterosuperiorly. If the presence of the artery within the partition is not recognized, it can be injured during endoscopic sinus surgery. The right anterior ethmoidal foramen is also seen (*asterisk*).

Local digital trauma to the nose is the most common cause of epistaxis, usually resulting in mild hemorrhage of the anterior nasal septum. Mucosal dryness can also predispose an individual to bleeding from this same area. Mucosal dryness can be due to turbulent airflow, caused by septal deviation or spurs, and low humidity. Epistaxis is more frequent during the winter months, presumably because of the lower humidity during that time. Intranasal corticosteroids can be a cause of mucosal bleeding. Patients should be counseled on proper application, directing the spray laterally to avoid direct application to the septum. Traumatic nasal bone fracture or septal fracture can result in significant acute epistaxis. Bleeding may recur or be delayed following maxillofacial trauma because of posttraumatic aneurysm of the septal vasculature. Rhinosinusitis may be a coexisting factor, particularly in children, and may lead to increased inflammation, nose blowing, or, potentially, digital trauma, resulting in epistaxis.

Systemic factors frequently contribute to severe uncontrollable epistaxis. Von Willebrand's disease and hemophilia are inherited coagulopathies and must be considered with a history of significant bleeding from minor wounds or severe bruising. Thrombocytopenia with a platelet counts of less than $20,000/mm^3$ can make controlling epistaxis challenging. Hematologic malignancies can produce a similar coagulopathy because of poor platelet production. Similarly, chemotherapy regimens can produce thrombocytopenia. Chronic alcohol intake, aspirin and other nonsteroidal anti-inflammatory medication usage, and renal failure affect platelet function, despite normal counts. The role of hypertension is debated and no clear independent association has been firmly established as a lone factor in epistaxis. However, hypertension may make controlling a bleed more difficult. Osler-Weber-Rendu disease (hereditary hemorrhagic telangiecta-sia) is an autosomal dominant disease that results in fragile telangiectasias and arteriovenous malformations that can also cause significant recurrent bleeding.

Anticoagulant medication use should be ascertained during evaluation. The use of coumadin, enoxaparin, and heparin all alter the coagulation cascade. Aspirin and other nonsteroidal anti-inflammatory drugs are com-monly used medications that affect platelet function. It is also important to inquire about alternative medicines. Garlic, ginkgo, and ginseng (the "3 Gs") are known to inhibit platelet function specifically by affecting aggre-gation. A coagulation panel should be checked on admission in anticoagu-lated patients, and reversal of the anticoagulant should be considered.

Any individual with recurrent bleeding and a lack of other systemic factors should be evaluated for neoplasia, especially when the bleeding is unilateral. Juvenile nasal angiofibroma is an uncommon tumor that selectively affects teenage boys. Other common nasal neoplasia include papillomas, hemangi-omas, squamous cell carcinomas, esthesioneuroblastomas, melanomas, and adenocarcinomas. These lesions typically result in recurrent epistaxis which is associated with nasal obstruction. Patients with this history should undergo nasal endoscopy and radiologic imaging to rule out neoplasia.

Evaluation

Once confirmation of hemodynamic stability and airway patency is complete, a directed history can quickly identify most of the factors contrib-uting to a severe nosebleed. Laterality of the nosebleed, amount of blood loss, severity, and duration should be ascertained. The presence of nasal obstruc-tion may indicate a neoplasm, especially with recurrent bleeding from the same side. If the nosebleed is traumatic in nature, one should consider other associated injuries. Attention must be given to other medical conditions, medications, alcohol use, and a history of severe nosebleeds or easy bruising. A family history of bleeding should also be investigated. Laboratory studies should be dictated by the history, physical examination, and severity of the bleeding and may include hematologic, coagulation, renal, and hepatic indices.

The examination seeks not only to rule out predisposing factors, such as telangiectasias or neoplasm but also to define precisely the source of bleed-ing. Epistaxis is typically classified as either anterior or posterior. These clas-sifications do not have a defined dividing line between them; instead, the definition is an operational one. Anterior epistaxis has traditionally been defined as bleeding controlled through anterior rhinoscopy or anterior nasal packing, whereas posterior epistaxis is bleeding not easily visible anteriorly or that which is controlled only through posterior packing. Recent advances in endoscopy and endoscopic ligation/cauterization techniques blur the lines between these two divisions. It may be more appropriate to define anterior epistaxis as bleeding arising from the more anterior vessels (anterior ethmoid artery, superior labial artery branches) and posterior epistaxis as bleeding arising from the more posterior vessels (sphenopalatine and posterior ethmoidal arteries). Although these definitions have a significant "gray area" because of anastomotic networks, such a classification helps define which treatment methods will likely be necessary.

The examination begins with anterior rhinoscopy, which should identify the most common locations for anterior bleeds and can also be performed easily in most children. Significant hemorrhage will require suction, a light source, and a nasal speculum. If no anterior source is identified, a nasal endoscope can be used to visualize the remainder of the nasal cavity. Attention should be paid to mucosal lesions or submucous masses within the middle meatus and nasopharynx. Commonly, multiple small abrasions are encountered in the nasal cavity, which is typically the result of previous attempts at control of the bleeding by other care providers. Topical vasoconstriction with oxymetazoline or phenylephrine mixed with a topical anesthetic such as lidocaine or pontocaine will enhance the examination and slow some of the bleeding. Suction may also be necessary, in a cooperative patient, for visualization. Care must be taken when manipulating clots in the nasopharynx, because they may be dislodged into the hypopharynx, impacting the airway.

Another useful adjunct for anatomic diagnosis during significant posterior bleeding is a transpalatal injection of the SPA where it enters the nasal cavity [6]. A 25-gauge needle is bent at 2.5 cm and inserted transorally into the greater palatine foramen to the bend. After withdrawing slightly to ensure the needle is not within a vessel, 1.5 mL of a 1:100,000 epinephrine solution is then injected slowly [7]. This vasoconstrictive injection will slow bleeding from the SPA branches, effectively making the diagnosis of "posterior epistaxis." Moreover, bleeding will usually slow substantially or even stop, typically allowing endoscopy to find the exact bleeding source. Quality endoscopy helps establish the bleeding location, which is essential in determining an appropriate treatment plan.

Treatment options

Treatment approaches vary, based on the severity and location of the bleeding, the predisposing or underlying factors, and the experience of the treating physician. Hemodynamic stability and intravenous access should be assured for patients seen emergently for epistaxis. Depending on the severity of the bleeding, assessing for anemia and cross-matching for possible transfusion may also be warranted.

Immediate medical treatment aims to stem the bleeding for both anterior and posterior bleeds and is often used initially to improve visualization during the physical examination. Topical vasoconstrictors are the first step in the management of any nosebleed. Topical 1% phenylephrine or 0.05% oxymetazoline are both commonly used agents for this purpose. Topical vasoconstrictors may be combined with a topical anesthetic agent, such as 2% to 4% lidocaine, to facilitate nasal endoscopy or topical treatment.

Anterior epistaxis

Cauterization can be used for anterior bleeds if an accessible bleeding site is identified either with anterior rhinoscopy or endoscopy. Chemical and electric cauterizations are commonly used and one or both of these methods can control most minor episodes of epistaxis. Silver nitrate sticks can be applied to the topically anesthetized nasal septum with minimum discomfort. The silver precipitates and is reduced to neutral silver metal. This reaction releases reactive oxygen species to coagulate tissue, which is most useful for minor bleeds but may be inadequate with more severe bleeds because the blood flow will wash away the silver nitrate before it can act. Cauterization should be limited to one side of the nasal septum, or separated by 4 to 6 weeks to avoid septal perforation [8].

Electric cauterization is useful for more aggressive bleeding of the anterior nasal septum. The nose must first be anesthetized using injected local anesthesia. It is important to anesthetize bilaterally because the electric current is transmitted through the septum and may cause significant discomfort. Again, conservative cauterization will avoid septal perforation. This cauterization can be done relatively easily for anterior bleeding sites; however, more posterior sites may require endoscopic visualization.

Laser cauterization has a limited role in the control of epistaxis. The most common application is for patients who have chronic epistaxis secondary to hereditary hemorrhagic telangiectasia. The telangiectasias can be electively controlled with laser photocoagulation; potassium-titanyl-phosphate or CO_2 lasers are used most frequently. Lasers have little role in the treatment of acute epistaxis.

Failure of cauterization or medical management leads a clinician to consider packing as the next treatment option. Many different types of packs have been developed over the years, including absorbable, nonabsorbable, anterior, and posterior packs. The otolaryngologist must be familiar with the different packing options available.

Common absorbable materials used for anterior packing include oxidized cellulose and gelatin foam. Oxidized cellulose (eg, Surgicel) and gelatin foams (eg, Gelfoam) encourage platelet aggregation and, when placed in the nose, they not only tamponade the bleeding but also protect the mucosa from further desiccation or trauma to promote healing. Another product combines thrombin with gelatin to produce a slurry (eg, Floseal) that is applied relatively easily to the nose. The benefits of thrombin-gelatin products are ease of application, patient comfort, and conformity to the irregular contours of the nasal cavity. Brisk arterial bleeding may not be as effectively controlled by these products; however, most other bleeding is treated adequately. Mathiasen [9] showed in a prospective randomized controlled study that thrombin-gelatin is easier to use, less painful, and more effective in emergency room patients for initial control of epistaxis. However, thrombin-gelatin is more expensive than traditional packing. Conversely, the use of thrombin-gelatin may obviate otolaryngology consultation or the need for packing removal.

Various nonabsorbable packing materials are available, including inflatable balloons, carboxymethylcellulose sponges, calcium alginate, or petroleum jelly–impregnated gauze. It is important to be familiar with multiple options for anterior packing. The drawback of anterior packing is the need for removal and the discomfort associated with placement and removal. Patients who have nasal packing should also be placed on antibiotics to avoid toxic shock syndrome. Coating the packs with antibiotic ointment is often recommended but no evidence exists to demonstrate any reduction in infectious complications. Packs are generally left in for 1 to 5 days based on physician preference, response of the patient, risk factors, state of coagulopathy, and severity of initial bleed.

Failure to control anterior bleeding with packing or cautery may necessitate ligation of the ethmoidal vessels. The anterior ethmoid artery cannot be embolized angiographically because of the risk of blindness or stroke. The traditional approach for surgical ligation is through a Lynch incision. The periosteum is raised off the lacrimal crest and posteriorly into the orbit. The anterior ethmoid artery is located 24 mm posterior to the lacrimal crest, between the periorbita and the lamina papyracea. The artery is then clipped or coagulated using bipolar electrocauterization. A transnasal endoscopic approach through the lamina papyracea has recently been described, although it is more technically challenging and the risks to the orbit and skull base may outweigh the benefit of avoiding an external incision [10]. Endoscopic bipolar cauterization of the bleeding site may also be useful in a well-anesthetized and vasoconstricted nose. Endoscopes or microscopes can be helpful through the external approach, providing improved magnification and lighting [11]. The posterior ethmoid artery, when present, may also contribute to epistaxis. The surgeon must balance the risk of persistent bleeding with the risk of injury to the optic nerve, 6 mm posterior to the posterior ethmoidal artery [12]. If a prominent vessel is not seen 12 to 14 mm posterior to the anterior ethmoidal artery, a posterior ethmoid artery may not be present and termination of the exploration is probably warranted.

Posterior epistaxis

Posterior bleeds require different methods for adequate control. Bleeding in the posterior nasal cavity, as noted above, most likely originates from the SPA, although the posterior ethmoidal artery may rarely be a source. Diagnosis and localization can be difficult at times, even with endoscopic evaluation. Because of the frequent severity of the bleeding and the relative inaccessibility of the source, medical treatments, standard packing, and silver nitrate cauterization have limited roles in posterior nasal bleeding. The main methods of treatment include endoscopic electric cauterization, posterior packing, embolization, and surgical arterial ligation.

Thornton and colleagues [13] recently published a series of 43 patients in whom posterior bleeding could not be controlled with conservative measures. They successfully cauterized posterior bleeding sites in 81%. The most common site of bleeding was on the lateral nasal wall. More than one third of their patients had bleeding from the lateral aspect of the posterior portion of the turbinates. These locations may make electrocauterization technically challenging. Posterior nasal cauterization often requires general anesthesia and a thorough examination with rigid endoscopes.

Posterior packing is not as commonly used as anterior packing and involves more risk. A posterior pack may be an emergent temporizing procedure before other surgical therapy. Posterior packs are available commercially; most of these involve an anterior balloon and a posterior balloon with separate ports for differential inflation pressures. The posterior balloon abuts the choana and fills the posterior nasal cavity. These posterior packs can be painful and put significant pressure on the septum and posterior portion of the turbinates. If a double balloon pack is not available, an (some argue preferable) alternative is to use a Foley catheter (12 or 14 F) combined with an anterior pack. After the balloon is tested, the Foley is placed into the nasal cavity, the balloon is inflated (5–10 mL saline), and the catheter is pulled anterior until the balloon lodges in the choana. Inflation of the balloon is adjusted until the soft palate is not displaced, to prevent soft palate necrosis. Other packing material (eg, petroleum-impregnated gauze or a commercial anterior pack) can then be placed anterior to the Foley catheter to fill the remainder of the nasal cavity and secure additional pressure on the bleeding point. The Foley catheter must be secured at the nasal sill to maintain pressure and to avoid posterior migration into the pharynx. Padding should be used to protect the ala and columella, both of which are at risk for pressure necrosis.

Complications from anterior and posterior packs include ulcerations, septal perforation, sinusitis, synechiae, hypoxemia, and arrhythmias. Posterior packing can lead to alar, columellar, or palatal necrosis. The posterior pack may also cause apnea and hypoxia, with possible dysrhythmia. The apnea and hypoxia associated with posterior packing has previously been ascribed to stimulation of the nasopulmonary or "diving" reflex. Such a reflex pathway has never been firmly established and it is more likely that this phenomenon is a result of obstructive sleep apnea. Patients who have posterior packing should be admitted for inpatient observation, with pulse oximetry and supplemental oxygen supplied as needed. Care should be taken in individuals with a history of cardiopulmonary disease.

Posterior packing is successful in 70% of patients [2]. If a posterior pack is not successful, repositioning can be attempted because the packs tend to migrate anteriorly. The modest success rate, need for a monitored hospital stay, significant patient discomfort, and risk of cardiopulmonary events limit the enthusiasm for packing as a treatment option for posterior epistaxis.

Embolization for epistaxis was first performed by Sokoloff in 1974. Since then, embolization has become an accepted treatment for posterior epistaxis, where available. Common embolization targets include the IMA and facial artery. These vessels can be embolized with various materials, including cyanoacrylate glue, polyvinyl alcohol sponges, metal coils, or gelatin foam. Bilateral IMA ligation is often used for cases in which the exact source is unidentifiable. Success rates have ranged from 79% to 96% in multiple studies [14]. However, complication rates as high as 24% have been reported. Complications from embolization include rebleeding, stroke, blindness, facial numbness, skin sloughing, carotid artery dissection, and groin hematoma. Embolization therapy has been evaluated with regard to cost in several studies. Miller and colleagues [15] showed that embolization was twice as costly as modern surgical treatment for recurrent epistaxis. Another detractor of embolization is its inability to control bleeding from the ethmoidal arteries. Many institutions may not have capable interventionalists available to embolize posterior bleeds. In this situation, if packing fails to control the bleeding, surgical treatment may become necessary.

Once the decision to proceed with surgical therapy is entertained, one must consider which arteries to target. This decision is based on physical examination, endoscopy, history, and thorough knowledge of the vascular supply of the nose. For persistent posterior bleeding, ligation of the IMA has historically been used [16]. The approach is similar to that used for a Caldwell-Luc operation, with access through the posterior maxillary wall into the pterygomaxillary fossa. The IMA is then identified and can be clipped or cauterized with bipolar electrocauterization. Known complications include sinusitis, facial and gum numbness, and oroantral fistula [17]. Difficulty in identifying the IMA in the pterygomaxillary fossa, and the potential for anastomoses distal to the ligation, such as in the descending palatine artery, may explain the failures of this approach, which are reported to be as high as 40% [18].

Over time, surgical treatment of posterior epistaxis has advanced from ligation of the external carotid artery to transantral ligation of the IMA, as described above, and, more recently, to endoscopic ligation of the SPA. The SPA is the end artery that supplies a major portion of the nasal cavity; therefore, ligation here is more successful than other surgical approaches [19].

Transnasal endoscopic sphenopalatine artery ligation (TESPAL) was first described in 1992 by Budrovich and Saetti [20]. The procedure can be performed under general or local anesthesia [21]. The nose is adequately decongested topically, and the SPA is injected with lidocaine with epinephrine through the greater palatine foramen, as described above. A 0°, 4-mm telescope is used to visualize the posterior portion of the middle turbinate and its attachment to the lateral nasal wall. More local anesthetic can be injected into this portion of the nose to dampen further bleeding. Next, a 10- to 20-mm incision is made vertically 5 mm anterior to the attachment of the middle turbinate. A mucosal flap is raised posteriorly until the crista ethmoidalis is reached. The SPA enters the nose posterior to this consistent landmark (Fig. 2) [22]. The artery is identified and may be dissected free from the maxillary division and nasopalatine nerve. Resection of the crista ethmoidalis with a Kerrison punch may improve visualization. The SPA is then clipped or cauterized as it enters the nasal cavity close to the lateral wall (Fig. 3), which insures inclusion of any posterior branches that may diverge early. Following ligation or cauterization, the artery is divided and the area explored posteriorly for 2 to 3 mm to ensure no other vessels remain, the flap is replaced, and the patient is observed. Further packing is not required and results are 87% to 100% control.

Complications reported with TESPAL include palatal numbness, sinusitis, decreased lacrimation, and septal perforation. Necrosis of the inferior turbinate has also been reported following this procedure. No major complications have been reported. The procedure uses standard endoscopic sinus surgery equipment, which is available to most otolaryngologists. TESPAL can also be combined with anterior ethmoid artery ligation if a superior bleeding source is clinically suspected. Given its high success rates, this procedure has become our treatment of choice for posterior epistaxis.

The timing of TESPAL or other surgical modalities is controversial. Early intervention may result in a shorter hospital course, improved control of bleeding, avoidance of the discomfort of packing, and ultimately, less cost, as shown by Miller and colleagues. Similarly, Miller and colleagues

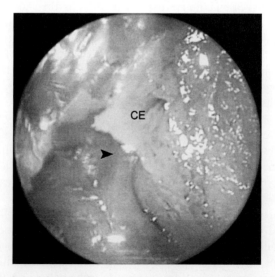

Fig. 2. Ligation of the left SPA. The artery (*arrowhead*) emerges from the sphenopalatine foramen immediately posterior to the crista ethmoidalis (CE). Zero-degree endoscope.

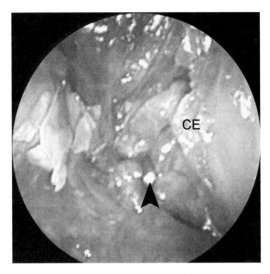

Fig. 3. Ligation of the left SPA. A single clip (*arrowhead*) has been applied to the SPA. Zero-degree endoscope. CE, crista ethmoidalis.

[23] showed that surgical treatment was less costly than packing when used as primary treatment. Ultimately, early consideration of TESPAL should be given in situations in which severe posterior epistaxis is refractory to conservative management. At the authors' institution, TESPAL is performed as the primary modality for patients presenting with posterior epistaxis, typically under local anesthesia with mild sedation, and with patients usually going home without an inpatient hospital stay.

Once epistaxis is controlled, conservative measures may help avoid recurrent bleeding due to local factors. Nasal saline washes and water-soluble ointments assist in humidification of the nasal mucosal, and promote healing. Saline or other moisturizing nasal sprays may also be used. Humidified air, especially for patients using nasal cannula oxygen, may also further improve the local conditions within the nose. Control of inflammation within the nose may be helpful to avoid further irritation or manipulation of the nose.

Summary

Epistaxis is a common problem that ranges from a minor nuisance to a life-threatening emergency. Multiple modalities exist to treat anterior and posterior bleeding and sometimes more than one treatment must be used. Otolaryngologists must be prepared to deal with severe or refractory bleeding through the use of medications, packing materials, and radiologic or surgical interventions. Identifying the likely source of the bleeding based on a thorough knowledge of the vascular anatomy increases the likelihood of successful treatment.

References

[1] Weiss NS. Relation of high blood pressure to headache, epistaxis, and selected other symptoms. The United States Health Examination Survey of Adults. N Engl J Med 1972;287: 631–3.

[2] Massick D, Tobin EJ. Epistaxis. In: Cummings CW, Haughey BH, Thomas JR, et al, editors. Cummings otolaryngology: head and neck surgery. Philadelphia: Mosby; 2005. p. 942–61.

[3] Floreani SR, Nair SB, Switajewski MC, et al. Endoscopic anterior ethmoidal artery ligation: a cadaver study. Laryngoscope 2006;116:1263–7.

[4] Tan LK, Calhoun KH. Epistaxis. Med Clin North Am 1999;83:43–56.

[5] Wormald PJ. Epistaxis. In: Bailey BJ, Calhoun KH, Derkay C, et al, editors. Head and neck surgery - otolaryngology. Philadelphia: Lippincott Williams & Wilkins; 2006. p. 505–14.

[6] Orlandi RR, Lanza DC. Is nasal packing necessary following endoscopic sinus surgery? Laryngoscope 2004;114(9):1541–4.

[7] Douglas R, Wormald PJ. Pterygopalatine fossa infiltration through the greater palatine foramen: where to bend the needle. Laryngoscope 2006;116(7):1255–7.

[8] Hanif J, Tasca RA, Frosh A, et al. Silver nitrate: histological effects of cautery on epithelial surfaces with varying contact times. Clin Otolaryngol Allied Sci 2003;28(4):368–70.

[9] Mathiasen RA, Cruz R. Prospective, randomized, controlled clinical trial of a novel matrix hemostatic sealant in patients with acute anterior epistaxis. Laryngoscope 2005;115(5): 899–902.

[10] Pletcher SD, Metson R. Endoscopic ligation of the anterior ethmoid artery. Laryngoscope 2007;117(2):378–81.

[11] Douglas SA, Gupta D. Endoscopic assisted external approach anterior ethmoidal artery ligation for the management of epistaxis. J Laryngol Otol 2003;117(2):132–3.

[12] Brouz D, Charakidas A, Androulakis M, et al. Traumatic optic neuropathy after posterior ethmoidal artery ligation for epistaxis. Otolaryngol Head Neck Surg 2002;126(3):323–5.

[13] Thornton MA, Mahesh BN, Lang J. Posterior epistaxis: identification of common bleeding sites. Laryngoscope 2005;115(4):588–90.

[14] Smith TP. Embolization in the external carotid artery. J Vasc Interv Radiol 2006;17(12): 1897–912.

[15] Miller TR, Stevens ES, Orlandi RR. Economic analysis of the treatment of posterior epistaxis. Am J Rhinol 2005;19:79–82.

[16] Pope LE, Hobbs CG. Epistaxis: an update on current management. Postgrad Med J 2005;81: 309–14.

[17] Morgan MK, Aldren CP. Oroantral fistula: a complication of transantral ligation of the internal maxillary artery for epistaxis. J Laryngol Otol 1997;111(5):468–70.

[18] Srinivasan V, Sherman IW, O'Sullivan G. Surgical management of intractable epistaxis: audit of results. J Laryngol Otol 2000;114(9):697–700.

[19] Kumar S, Shetty A, Rockey J, et al. Contemporary surgical treatment of epistaxis. What is the evidence for sphenopalatine artery ligation? Clin Otolaryngol Allied Sci 2003;28(4): 360–3.

[20] Budrovich R, Saetti R. Microscopic and endoscopic ligature of the sphenopalatine artery. Laryngoscope 1992;102(12):1391–4.

[21] Orlandi RR. Endoscopic sphenopalatine artery ligation. Op Tech Otolaryngol Head Neck Surg 2001;12(2):98–100.

[22] Bolger WE, Borgie RC, Melder P. The role of the crista ethmoidalis in endoscopic sphenopalatine artery ligation. Am J Rhinol 1999;13(2):81–6.

[23] Klotz DA, Winkle MR, Richmon J, et al. Surgical management of posterior epistaxis: a changing paradigm. Laryngoscope 2002;112:1577–82.

ELSEVIER
SAUNDERS

Otolaryngol Clin N Am
41 (2008) 537–549

OTOLARYNGOLOGIC
CLINICS
OF NORTH AMERICA

Malignant Otitis Externa

Matthew J. Carfrae, MD, Bradley W. Kesser, MD*

*Department of Otolaryngology – Head and Neck Surgery, Division of Otology-Neurotology,
University of Virginia Health System, Box 800713, 1 Hospital Drive, Old Medical School,
2nd Floor, Charlottesville, VA 22908, USA*

Malignant (necrotizing) otitis externa (MOE) was first described as a case of progressive *Pseudomonas* osteomyelitis in the temporal bone of a patient who had diabetes nearly a half century ago [1]. Chandler [2] published the first series of patients with progressive osteomyelitis of the temporal bone and termed the condition *malignant otitis externa*. Other authors have advocated using the term *necrotizing* otitis externa to reflect the fact that the process is not neoplastic [3]. *Skull base osteomyelitis* perhaps most accurately describes the pathophysiology of the disease process and has been used to indicate infection that has spread to the skull base, beyond the external auditory canal [3]. Although perhaps less precise, *malignant otitis externa* has been used most extensively in the literature and common vernacular, and will be the term used in this article.

Before effective antibiotic regimens, MOE was frequently fatal, with mortality rates of nearly 50% [2]. Originally managed surgically, MOE is now effectively treated with antibiotics in most cases, with surgery reserved for biopsy and local debridement. Prompt identification and diagnosis of MOE and appropriate culture-directed therapy can prevent serious complications and mortality.

Epidemiology

Diabetes mellitus remains the most important associated condition. Although only 65% of subjects had diabetes in a recent review of 46 cases of malignant otitis externa [4], the prevalence of diabetes in MOE is more commonly 90% to 100% of patients [2,5–8]. Any condition causing immunosuppression, including HIV/AIDS [9,10], chemotherapy-induced aplasia, refractory anemia, chronic leukemia, lymphoma, splenectomy, neoplasia,

---

* Corresponding author.
E-mail address: bwk2n@virginia.edu (B.W. Kesser).

0030-6665/08/$ - see front matter © 2008 Elsevier Inc. All rights reserved.
doi:10.1016/j.otc.2008.01.004   *oto.theclinics.com*

and renal transplantation, may predispose a patient to MOE [4,5]. As recognized in Chandler's [2] seminal review, however, patients who have diabetes (and especially elderly patients) are particularly vulnerable to MOE because of the associated endarteritis, microangiopathy, and small vessel obliteration, which, coupled with the ability of *Pseudomonas* to invade vessel walls and cause a vasculitis with thrombosis and coagulation necrosis of surrounding tissue, underlies the pathophysiology of this disease.

Patients who have HIV-associated MOE are younger than the average patient who has diabetes. MOE should be suspected in all patients who have HIV and otitis externa that does not improve with appropriate therapy. MOE in patients who have HIV may lack typical granulation tissue along the floor of the external auditory canal (EAC) [10]. Fungal MOE is found in patients who have HIV more commonly than in those who have diabetes, particularly patients who have severe AIDS [11]. Fungal MOE often originates in the middle ear or mastoid in contrast to pseudomonal MOE. *Pseudomonas* infections in HIV occur with CD4 levels less than 100 cells/mm and *Aspergillus*-associated MOE with CD4 counts less than 50 cells/mm [9].

Although rare, MOE has been reported in children who have diabetes and other immunocompromised states, including IgG subclass deficiency [12], IgA deficiency [13], acute monocytic leukemia [14], iatrogenic neutropenia secondary to induction chemotherapy for acute lymphoblastic leukemia [15], and bone marrow transplantation [16]. Compared with adults, diabetes is not as common a comorbidity in children (21% in one review [14]) as are other immunocompromised states.

The course of MOE in children has an acute onset, with more toxic initial symptoms of fever, malaise, and leukocytosis. Although one review reported a lower incidence of facial nerve paralysis in children [14], another cited a higher incidence earlier in the course of the disease because of the less-developed mastoid process and closer proximity of the facial nerve and stylomastoid foramen to the EAC [17]. Facial paralysis has no prognostic significance to overall recovery, because both studies agree that children generally have a more favorable prognosis than adults [14,17]. Prognosis for facial nerve recovery in children is poorer, however [14]. *P aeruginosa* is also the most common causative agent in children. Complications in children include necrosis of the tympanic membrane [17], stenosis of the EAC, auricular deformity, and sensorineural and conductive hearing loss [14,17]. Most pediatric cases resolve with several weeks of intravenous antibiotics, although longer courses can be required [18]. Quinolones are generally avoided in children because of damage to weight-bearing joints in juvenile animal studies. However, ciprofloxacin has been successfully used to treat resistant MOE in a child after other intravenous therapy failed [14].

Pathophysiology

MOE affects immunocompromised individuals; its presentation in an otherwise healthy individual should prompt an investigation for diabetes mellitus or other immunodeficiency. MOE originates as a soft tissue infection of the EAC. Water irrigation for cerumen disimpaction in elderly patients who have diabetes is a proposed inciting event [19]. Histologic studies of the EAC show inflammation of the epidermis with acute and chronic inflammatory reaction in the dermis [20]. Patients who have diabetes show poor chemotaxis and phagocytosis of polymorphonuclear leukocytes, monocytes, and macrophages, leading to susceptibility to *P aeruginosa* infection [21,22]. Another contributing factor may be the higher pH of cerumen in individuals who have diabetes [23].

Infection from the EAC spreads to the skull base through the fissures of Santorini, small perforations in the cartilaginous portion of the EAC found along the floor of the canal. Once out of the canal, infection spreads medially to the tympanomastoid suture, and along venous canals and fascial planes. The compact bone of the skull base becomes replaced with granulation tissue, leading to bone destruction. Progressive spread of infection to skull base foramina causes cranial neuropathies. The most commonly involved nerve is the facial nerve because of the proximity of the stylomastoid foramen to the EAC. Nerves of the jugular foramen are the next most commonly affected. As disease spreads more medially, petrous apex involvement can affect the abducens and trigeminal nerves and, more medially, the optic nerve [24]. Spread of infection to the sigmoid sinus can lead to septic thrombosis of the sigmoid sinus and internal jugular vein; meningitis and cerebral abscess may also complicate MOE [3,25]. Skull base osteomyelitis can also spread to the contralateral side and include the cervical spine [26]. Finally, extracranial spread of infection may involve the infratemporal fossa, parotid, and neck, leading to involvement of surrounding structures and abscess formation. The otic capsule is typically spared and middle ear involvement is usually a late finding [2,3].

Microbiology

In most cases, the causative agent of MOE is *Pseudomonas aeruginosa*, which is a gram-negative obligate aerobe not normally found in the EAC. This organism will colonize the EAC in a moist environment or after trauma and is only a pathogen in the absence of effective host defenses. It also commonly causes benign acute otitis externa (swimmer's ear). Conditions leading to more invasive MOE must also involve impaired host immunity to allow the organism to spread out of the external canal. More virulent *Pseudomonas* species contain a mucoid surface layer that protects the bacterium from phagocytosis. They also produce lytic enzymes, including endotoxin, collagenase, and elastase, causing a necrotizing vasculitis and endarteritis that enable invasion of surrounding tissue. Other bacteria, including *Staphylococcus aureus* [27], *S epidermidis* [28], *Proteus mirabilis* [29], *Klebsiella oxytoca* [30], and *P cepacia* [31], have also been reported to cause MOE, although these organisms may have been colonizers and not true pathogens.

Fungal pathogens can also cause MOE, particularly in immunocompromised patients who are not diabetic, including those who have HIV/AIDS [25]. The most common fungal organism is *Aspergillus fumigatus* [32,33], although other species have been isolated, including *A flavus* [34,35], *A niger* (in a patient who was immunocompetent [36] and one who was diabetic [37]), and *Scedosporium apiospermum* (in a patient who had end-stage AIDS [11]). The possibility of fungal MOE must be considered if a patient who has classic signs and symptoms of MOE is unresponsive to appropriate antimicrobial therapy and cultures have been negative. Fungal MOE should also be considered and cultures retaken in patients who do well initially on antimicrobial therapy but experience recrudescence [34]. Several studies point out the clinical differences between bacterial and fungal MOE (Table 1).

Finally, the diagnosis and treatment of MOE in the absence of an identifiable pathogen (culture-negative specimen) has been described. These studies diagnosed MOE based on clinical history, signs and symptoms, biopsy to rule out malignancy, markedly elevated erythrocyte sedimentation rate (ESR), and imaging studies, such as CT and radionuclide (gallium and technetium bone) scanning [8,38]. Previous treatment with oral or topical antibiotics before evaluation and wound culture may be responsible for this scenario, because many patients had already experienced failed response to a short course of oral ciprofloxacin and various topical antibiotic preparations before undergoing otolaryngologic evaluation. Treatment included intravenous ceftazidime (aztreonam for penicillin allergic patients), high-dose oral ciprofloxacin (750 mg twice daily), and topical aminoglycoside–steroid drops [8].

Clinical presentation

Typical patients who have MOE are elderly individuals who have diabetes and severe, unremitting otalgia, aural fullness, otorrhea, and hearing loss. Otalgia in these patients may be worse at night and more severe than what is usually associated with otitis externa. Hearing loss is conductive in nature. Headache, temporomandibular joint pain, and decreased oral intake secondary to trismus may also be present. Patients may provide a history of minor ear canal trauma associated with irrigation or cleaning. Many patients will have already taken short courses of oral antibiotics or been prescribed topical antibiotic drops. This antecedent history of antimicrobial therapy should not deter clinicians from pursuing and diagnosing MOE (and ruling out malignancy).

On examination, purulent otorrhea with a swollen, tender external auditory canal are hallmarks. Skin of the concha may be erythematous and tender. Granulation tissue or exposed bone is frequently seen on the floor of the canal at the bony–cartilaginous junction. Usually the tympanic membrane and middle ear appear healthy and uninvolved if not obstructed by granulation tissue or polyp in the canal. Periaural lymphadenopathy may

Table 1
Clinical and microscopic differences between bacterial and fungal malignant otitis externa

Etiologic agent	Age	Diabetes	Immunosuppression	Granulation tissue	Middle ear/mastoid involvement	Histology
Bacteria (*Pseudomonas aeruginosa*)	Older	Common	Common	+	−	Gram-negative rod
Fungus (*Aspergillus* spp)	Younger	Less common	More common, especially cellular immunity, AIDS	−	+	Branching septated hyphae; calcium oxalate crystals [36]

Abbreviations: +, present; −, absent.
Data from Refs. [34–36].

also be present. Associated cranial neuropathies are caused by spread of infection through the skull base. Involvement of the stylomastoid foramen will lead to facial paralysis in 25% of patients; less frequently, involvement of the jugular foramen leads to deficits in cranial nerves IX, X, and XI [7,12]. Fever and leukocytosis are frequently absent. Dural sinus thrombosis, meningitis, and cerebral abscess may also complicate MOE and are late findings that portend a grave prognosis. The diagnosis of MOE should be considered in all immunocompromised patients, especially those who have diabetes, who have external otitis and severe otalgia.

Diagnosis

The diagnosis of MOE relies on specific elements of the history and physical examination and laboratory and imaging studies. Findings of pain disproportionate to the examination, otorrhea, and granulation tissue along the floor of the ear canal at the bony–cartilaginous junction are usually the first nonspecific signs and symptoms of MOE. Differential diagnosis includes carcinoma of the ear canal, granulomatous diseases, Paget's disease, nasopharyngeal malignances, clival lesions, and fibrous dysplasia [25]. Carcinoma of the ear canal has similar clinical and radiologic findings, and biopsy is absolutely necessary to rule out this disease. Additionally, repeat biopsy and cultures are warranted to rule out an occult malignancy if inflammatory disease persists despite appropriate antibiotic therapy. Fever and leukocytosis are typically absent in adults who have MOE. ESR is always elevated and has been advocated as a nonspecific inflammatory marker for diagnosis and resolution of disease [39].

Even if patients have used antibiotic drops, cultures should be taken for aerobic, anaerobic, and fungal organisms and for bacterial sensitivity. Tissue biopsies should be sent to pathology to rule out malignancy and to microbiology for culture. Silver stain on histologic sections may identify fungal pathogens. Repeat cultures are necessary if the first set of cultures is negative, but withholding therapy until cultures are positive is not recommended.

No imaging modality provides adequate anatomic and physiologic detail sufficient to diagnose and follow MOE. CT is sensitive to bone erosion and decreased skull base density, a later finding in MOE (Fig. 1) [40,41]. CT scanning is also sensitive in diagnosing abscess formation and involvement of the mastoid, temporomandibular joint, infratemporal fossa, nasopharynx, petrous apex, and carotid canal. Demineralization of the skull base of 30% or greater is identifiable on CT scan, but because these changes persist despite resolution of disease, CT is therefore a poor choice for measuring treatment response. CT is also inadequate for showing intracranial extension and bone marrow involvement.

MRI better shows changes in soft tissue, particularly dural enhancement and involvement of medullary bone spaces [41]. The persistence of these radiographic changes despite resolution of disease also makes MRI

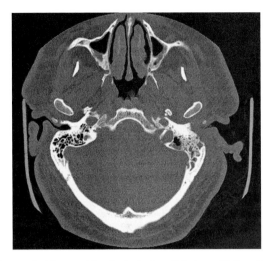

Fig. 1. Axial CT scan of a 63-year-old patient who has diabetes and left malignant otitis externa showing bony erosion of the posterior external auditory canal and mastoid cortex.

a poor study for determining disease resolution. Involvement of the retro-condylar fat pad on MRI has been proposed as an early diagnostic finding in patients being evaluated for MOE [42], but MRI is generally not recommended as a first-line diagnostic imaging modality (given its lower sensitivity for imaging bone erosion compared with CT).

Nuclear imaging has been a mainstay in the diagnosis and follow-up evaluation of patients who have MOE. Technetium Tc 99m methylene diphosphonate (MDP) scintigraphy (*bone scan*) is positive in almost 100% of MOE cases (Fig. 2). Technetium Tc 99m MDP radiotracer concentrates in areas with osteoblastic activity, as found in infection, trauma, and neoplasm. Given its high sensitivity, technetium Tc 99m MDP imaging allows earlier diagnosis of osteomyelitis than CT [43]. Sensitivity for MOE can be improved through identifying increased uptake between 4 and 24 hours postinjection [44]. However, technetium Tc 99m MDP scans are not specific for infection; they will also be positive in malignancy, hence the need to rule out malignancy with tissue biopsy. Technetium Tc 99m MDP bone scans remain positive indefinitely and are therefore not useful as markers of response to therapy or disease resolution.

Gallium Ga 67 citrate concentrates in areas of active inflammation through attaching to lactoferrin, which is present in large quantities in leukocytes, and through binding to transferrin and bacteria directly [45]. Gallium scans will be positive for soft tissue and bone infections (Fig. 3). Gallium uptake returns to normal after the infection has cleared, and several studies have suggested repeating gallium studies every 4 weeks to assess treatment response, and as a reliable test to stop treatment if negative [25,46]. Gallium scans have also proven useful in detecting recurrent disease

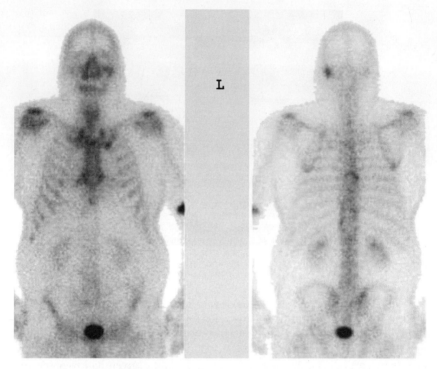

Fig. 2. Anterior and posterior views of technetium Tc 99m MDP bone scan of patient from Fig. 1 showing increased uptake in the left mastoid.

[26]. Both gallium and technetium Tc 99m MDP scans show poor anatomic resolution but are complementary in the diagnosis of MOE (Table 2).

Management

Successful management of MOE frequently requires collaboration with an endocrinologist, neurologist, radiologist, and infectious disease specialist.

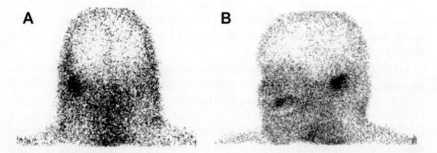

Fig. 3. Gallium scan of patient from Fig. 1 indicating increased inflammatory activity in the left mastoid region on posterior (A) and left lateral (B) views.

Table 2
Role of technetium, gallium, and CT scans in malignant otitis externa and malignancy

Condition	Gallium	Technetium	CT
Otitis externa	+	−	−
Malignant otitis externa (MOE)	+	+	May be (−)
Skull base osteomyelitis (SBO)	+	+	+
Recurrent MOE	(−) after treatment, then (+)	+	(+), if SBO
Resolved MOE	−	+	(+), if SBO
Malignancy	(−) in early disease, (+) with increasing growth	(−) in early disease, (+) with increasing bone involvement	(−) early in disease, (+) with increasing growth

Important principles of treatment include aggressive control of diabetes, reversal of acidosis, and improvement of immunocompetency, where possible. Although surgical intervention is no longer standard care for MOE, therapy does require biopsy and culture, and may require local debridement of granulation tissue and bony sequestration or drainage of associated abscess. Long-term antibiotic therapy is the mainstay of MOE treatment. Culture-directed therapy should always be the goal of treatment, and should be continued for at least 6 to 8 weeks. Previously, antipseudomonal penicillins and aminoglycosides were commonly used. This effective combination required parenteral administration and monitoring for ototoxicity and nephrotoxicity, especially in patients who had diabetes prone to chronic renal insufficiency.

Long-term monotherapy with oral ciprofloxacin (750 mg twice daily) has been proposed as the preferred initial antibiotic regimen [6]. Fluoroquinolones are active against P aeruginosa, penetrate bone well, have excellent oral bioavailability, and a less significant side effect profile compared with alternatives. Addition of rifampin, which does not affect the pharmacokinetics or bactericidal activity of ciprofloxacin, has also been suggested in MOE [39]. Newer-generation oral fluoroquinolone antibiotics other than ciprofloxacin may also be considered, but none has been reported in MOE.

Increasing incidence of pseudomonal resistance to ciprofloxacin has more recently been reported [5]. Resistance is related to widespread use of quinolones in the treatment of upper respiratory infections, topical preparations for otitis media and externa, and inadequate treatment courses in MOE. Berenholz and colleagues [5] found 33% P aeruginosa in MOE were resistant to ciprofloxacin. At the University of Virginia, resistance to P aeruginosa runs 20% in the outpatient setting. Avoidance of topical quinolones in noninvasive external ear infections, in favor of acidifying agents such as boric and acetic acid, has been recommended [5,19]. Use of topical antibiotics in MOE is controversial because these preparations only change bacterial flora of the EAC, making culture more difficult and introducing a potential source of antibiotic resistance without adding significant benefit [19,25].

Third-generation cephalosporins with antipseudomonal activity, such as ceftazidime, provide an alternative to ciprofloxacin in the treatment of MOE [5,47,48]. Ceftazidime requires parenteral administration, with resultant increased treatment cost and inconvenience to patients. Use of a concurrent aminoglycoside has also been recommended in resistant and complicated cases [49,50].

Amphotericin B is the most commonly used antifungal agent for fungal MOE [32–35], but alternatives have been sought given its toxicity. Liposomal amphotericin B is a lipid formulation of the drug with lower toxicity and equal efficacy. Oral itraconazole has also been used after a successful short course of amphotericin B [11].

Recurrence rates of 15% to 20% have been reported for MOE [26]. In this study, three elderly patients who had diabetes experienced recurrence of inadequately treated MOE, resulting in death in two patients and significant morbidity in the third. In all cases, inadequate length of treatment with resolution of symptoms preceded recurrence. Despite relief of symptoms, prolonged treatment of 6 to 8 weeks is recommended. Therapy can be discontinued once the ESR and gallium scans have normalized. Close follow-up is still necessary, because recurrence of MOE up to a year has been reported.

The role of hyperbaric oxygen (HBO) in managing MOE is not well established. HBO increases the partial pressure of oxygen, improving hypoxia and allowing greater oxidative killing of bacteria. Some authors have advocated its use in MOE for refractory skull base osteomyelitis [18,26,51,52] and intracranial involvement [53]. HBO requires daily treatments for several weeks and side effects include oxygen toxicity, barotrauma, and tympanic membrane perforation. A thorough review of the Cochrane Database, Medline, and Embase found no randomized controlled trials of HBO in MOE and concluded that no clear evidence exists to show the efficacy of HBO compared with antibiotic or surgical treatment [54].

Mortality from MOE has decreased from greater than 50% [2] to 0% to 15% [51]. Facial palsy has been suggested to signify poor prognosis, indicating the need for a longer course of treatment before recovery [4]. Poor prognostic factors include *Aspergillus* infection [4] and MRI findings of middle cranial fossa and foramen magnum dural enhancement [42]. In a recent series of 23 patients, cranial nerve involvement was not associated with poorer outcome, as was reported previously [7]. In this study, lower cranial nerve dysfunction exhibited good recovery, whereas facial nerve function improved but some dysfunction persisted despite adequate treatment. These results indicate that with current therapy, cranial nerve involvement does not preclude cure, although patients may have incomplete recovery of facial nerve function.

Summary

MOE should be suspected in immunocompromised patients (especially those who have diabetes) who have severe otalgia, purulent otorrhea, and granulation tissue or exposed bone in the external auditory canal. Prompt diagnosis with nuclear and CT imaging, biopsy to rule out malignancy, and culture (aerobic, anaerobic, and fungal) is essential. Antimicrobial therapy, generally starting with a high-dose oral quinolone, may avert complications of MOE, including cranial neuropathies and even death. Resolution of symptoms, especially pain, along with follow-up gallium scanning directs length of therapy, which should continue for at least 6 weeks.

Acknowledgments

The authors wish to thank Brian Williamson, MD, for assistance with the radiologic images and text.

References

[1] Meltzer PE, Kelemen G. Pyocutaneous osteomyelitis of the temporal bone, mandible, and zygoma. Laryngoscope 1959;169:1300–16.

[2] Chandler JR. Malignant external otitis. Laryngoscope 1968;78:1257–94.

[3] Nadol JB Jr. Histopathology of pseudomonas osteomyelitis of the temporal bone starting as malignant external otitis. Am J Otolaryngol 1980;1:359–71.

[4] Franco-Vidal V, Blanchet H, Bebear C, et al. Necrotizing external otitis: a report of 46 cases. Otol Neurotol 2007;28:771–3.

[5] Berenholz L, Katzenell U, Harell M. Evolving resistant pseudomonas to ciprofloxacin in malignant otitis externa. Laryngoscope 2002;112:1619–22.

[6] Levenson MJ, Parisier SC, Dolitsky J, et al. Ciprofloxacin: drug of choice in the treatment of malignant external otitis (MEO). Laryngoscope 1991;101:821–4.

[7] Mani N, Sudhoff H, Rajagopal S, et al. Cranial nerve involvement in malignant external otitis: implications for clinical outcome. Laryngoscope 2007;117:907–10.

[8] Djalilian HR, Shamloo B, Thakkar KH, et al. Treatment of culture-negative skull base osteomyelitis [see comment]. Otol Neurotol 2006;27:250–5.

[9] Hern JD, Almeyda J, Thomas DM, et al. Malignant otitis externa in HIV and AIDS. J Laryngol Otol 1996;110:770–5.

[10] Ress BD, Luntz M, Telischi FF, et al. Necrotizing external otitis in patients with AIDS. Laryngoscope 1997;107:456–60.

[11] Yao M, Messner AH. Fungal malignant otitis externa due to *Scedosporium apiospermum*. Ann Otol Rhinol Laryngol 2001;110:377–80.

[12] Castro R, Robinson N, Klein J, et al. Malignant external otitis and mastoiditis associated with an IgG4 subclass deficiency in a child. Del Med J 1990;62:1417–21.

[13] Paul AC, Justus A, Balraj A, et al. Malignant otitis externa in an infant with selective IgA deficiency: a case report. Int J Pediatr Otorhinolaryngol 2001;60:141–5.

[14] Sobie S, Brodsky L, Stanievich JF. Necrotizing external otitis in children: report of two cases and review of the literature. Laryngoscope 1987;97:598–601.

[15] Wolff LJ. Necrotizing otitis externa during induction therapy for acute lymphoblastic leukemia. Pediatrics 1989;84:882–5.

[16] Tezcan I, Tuncer AM, Yenicesu I, et al. Necrotizing otitis externa, otitis media, peripheral facial paralysis, and brain abscess in a thalassemic child after allogeneic BMT. Pediatr Hematol Oncol 1998;15:459–62.

[17] Rubin J, Yu VL, Stool SE. Malignant external otitis in children. J Pediatr 1988;113:965–70.

[18] Sreepada GS, Kwartler JA. Skull base osteomyelitis secondary to malignant otitis externa. Curr Opin Otolaryngol Head Neck Surg 2003;11:316–23.

[19] Rubin Grandis J, Branstetter BF 4th, Yu VL. The changing face of malignant (necrotising) external otitis: clinical, radiological, and anatomic correlations. Lancet Infect Dis 2004;4: 34–9.

[20] Bernheim J, Sade J. Histopathology of the soft parts in 50 patients with malignant external otitis. J Laryngol Otol 1989;103:366–8.

[21] Naghibi M, Smith RP, Baltch AL, et al. The effect of diabetes mellitus on chemotactic and bactericidal activity of human polymorphonuclear leukocytes. Diabetes Res Clin Pract 1987; 4:27–35.

[22] Geerlings SE, Hoepelman AI. Immune dysfunction in patients with diabetes mellitus (DM). FEMS Immunol Med Microbiol 1999;26:259–65.

[23] Driscoll PV, Ramachandrula A, Drezner DA, et al. Characteristics of cerumen in diabetic patients: a key to understanding malignant external otitis? Otolaryngol Head Neck Surg 1993;109:676–9.

[24] Holder CD, Gurucharri M, Bartels LJ, et al. Malignant external otitis with optic neuritis. Laryngoscope 1986;96:1021–3.

[25] Slattery WH, Brackmann DE. Skull base osteomyelitis: malignant otitis externa. Otolaryngol Clin North Am 1996;29:795–806.

[26] Singh A, Al Khabori M, Hyder MJ. Skull base osteomyelitis: diagnostic and therapeutic challenges in atypical presentation. Otolaryngol Head Neck Surg 2005;133:121–5.

[27] Bayardelle P, Jolivet-Granger M, Larochelle D. Staphylococcal malignant external otitis. Can Med Assoc J 1982;126:155–6.

[28] Barrow HN, Levenson MJ. Necrotizing 'malignant' external otitis caused by Staphylococcus epidermidis. Arch Otolaryngol Head Neck Surg 1992;118:94–6.

[29] Coser PL, Stamm AE, Lobo RC, et al. Malignant external otitis in infants. Laryngoscope 1980;90:312–6.

[30] Garcia Rodriguez JA, Montes Martinez I, Gomez Gonzalez JL, et al. A case of malignant external otitis involving Klebsiella oxytoca. Eur J Clin Microbiol Infect Dis 1992;11:75–7.

[31] Dettelbach MA, Hirsch BE, Weissman JL. Pseudomonas cepacia of the temporal bone: malignant external otitis in a patient with cystic fibrosis. Otolaryngol Head Neck Surg 1994;111:528–32.

[32] Cunningham M, Yu VL, Turner J, et al. Necrotizing otitis externa due to Aspergillus in an immunocompetent patient. Arch Otolaryngol Head Neck Surg 1988;114:554–6.

[33] Menachof MR, Jackler RK. Otogenic skull base osteomyelitis caused by invasive fungal infection. Otolaryngol Head Neck Surg 1990;102:285–9.

[34] Kountakis SE, Kemper JV Jr, Chang CY, et al. Osteomyelitis of the base of the skull secondary to Aspergillus. Am J Otolaryngol 1997;18:19–22.

[35] Stodulski D, Kowalska B, Stankiewicz C. Otogenic skull base osteomyelitis caused by invasive fungal infection: case report and literature review. Eur Arch Otorhinolaryngol 2006;263:1070–6.

[36] Shelton JC, Antonelli PJ, Hackett R. Skull base fungal osteomyelitis in an immunocompetent host. Otolaryngol Head Neck Surg 2002;126:76–8.

[37] Bellini C, Antonini P, Ermanni S, et al. Malignant otitis externa due to Aspergillus niger. Scand J Infect Dis 2003;35:284–8.

[38] Sie KC, Glenn MG, Hillel AH, et al. Osteomyelitis of the skull base, etiology unknown. Otolaryngol Head Neck Surg 1991;104:252–6.

[39] Rubin J, Stoehr G, Yu VL, et al. Efficacy of oral ciprofloxacin plus rifampin for treatment of malignant external otitis. Arch Otolaryngol Head Neck Surg 1989;115:1063–9.

[40] Meyers BR, Mendelson MH, Parisier SC, et al. Malignant external otitis. comparison of monotherapy vs combination therapy. Arch Otolaryngol Head Neck Surg 1987;113:974–8.

[41] Grandis JR, Curtin HD, Yu VL. Necrotizing (malignant) external otitis: prospective comparison of CT and MR imaging in diagnosis and follow-up. Radiology 1995;196:499–504.

[42] Kwon BJ, Han MH, Oh SH, et al. MRI findings and spreading patterns of necrotizing external otitis: is a poor outcome predictable? Clin Radiol 2006;61:495–504.

[43] Strashun AM, Nejatheim M, Goldsmith SJ. Malignant external otitis: early scintigraphic detection. Radiology 1984;150:541–5.

[44] Hardoff R, Gips S, Uri N, et al. Semiquantitative skull planar and SPECT bone scintigraphy in diabetic patients: differentiation of necrotizing (malignant) external otitis from severe external otitis. J Nucl Med 1994;35:411–5.

[45] Stokkel MP, Boot CN, van Eck-Smit BL. SPECT gallium scintigraphy in malignant external otitis: initial staging and follow-up. Case reports. Laryngoscope 1996;106:338–40.

[46] Parisier SC, Lucente FE, Som PM, et al. Nuclear scanning in necrotizing progressive "malignant" external otitis. Laryngoscope 1982;92:1016–9.

[47] Kimmelman CP, Lucente FE. Use of ceftazidime for malignant external otitis. Ann Otol Rhinol Laryngol 1989;98:721–5.

[48] Johnson MP, Ramphal R. Malignant external otitis: report on therapy with ceftazidime and review of therapy and prognosis. Rev Infect Dis 1990;12:173–80.

[49] Cunha BA. Pseudomonas aeruginosa: resistance and therapy. Semin Respir Infect 2002;17: 231–9.

[50] Kraus DH, Rehm SJ, Kinney SE. The evolving treatment of necrotizing external otitis. Laryngoscope 1988;98:934–9.

[51] Narozny W, Kuczkowski J, Stankiewicz C, et al. Value of hyperbaric oxygen in bacterial and fungal malignant external otitis treatment. Eur Arch Otorhinolaryngol 2006;263:680–4.

[52] Shupak A, Greenberg E, Hardoff R, et al. Hyperbaric oxygenation for necrotizing (malignant) otitis externa. Arch Otolaryngol Head Neck Surg 1989;115:1470–5.

[53] Davis JC, Gates GA, Lerner C, et al. Adjuvant hyperbaric oxygen in malignant external otitis. Arch Otolaryngol Head Neck Surg 1992;118:89–93.

[54] Phillips JS, Jones SE. Hyperbaric oxygen as an adjuvant treatment for malignant otitis externa. Cochrane Database Syst Rev 2005;2:CD004617.

ELSEVIER
SAUNDERS

Otolaryngol Clin N Am
41 (2008) 551–566

OTOLARYNGOLOGIC
CLINICS
OF NORTH AMERICA

Epiglottitis and Croup

Steven E. Sobol, MD, MSc[a,b,]*, Syboney Zapata, MD[a,b]

[a]*Department of Otolaryngology–Head and Neck Surgery, Emory University School
of Medicine, 1405 Clifton Road, Atlanta, GA 30322, USA*
[b]*Section of Otolaryngology, Children's Healthcare of Atlanta at Egleston,
2015 Uppergate Drive, NE, Atlanta, GA, USA*

Croup

Laryngotracheobronchitis (croup) is a viral-mediated inflammatory condition of the subglottic airway that typically affects children between age 6 months and 3 years. Before the modern era of pediatric airway management, croup was considered a major cause of morbidity and mortality in children. Reports dating back to the 1800s describe as much as a 100% mortality rate from diphtheric croup, for which the only management was tracheotomy to bypass the obstructed airway. Although not the first to attempt intubation for croup, Joseph O'Dwyer, an obstetrician from New York, is credited with developing the first set of instruments designed for endotracheal intubation of children who had croup in the 1880s. In his first series of 50 cases of children who had croup, the mortality rate was 76% after intubation, which was an improvement over the almost certain death from the disease alone during this era. By 1887, O'Dwyer's mortality rate was as low as 50% [1].

With the advent of modern techniques to support and secure the airway, mortality from croup has become a rarity in developed countries. Most children can be managed in the primary care setting, with even the most recalcitrant cases manageable without the need for a surgical airway intervention.

Pathogenesis

The subglottis is the region of the airway between the true vocal folds and the trachea. It is the narrowest point of the pediatric airway and the most common site of inflammatory conditions causing clinically significant

---

* Corresponding author. Department of Otolaryngology–Head and Neck Surgery, Emory University School of Medicine, 2015 Uppergate Drive, NE, Room 218, Atlanta, GA.
E-mail address: ssobol@emory.edu (S.E. Sobol).

0030-6665/08/$ - see front matter © 2008 Elsevier Inc. All rights reserved.
doi:10.1016/j.otc.2008.01.012   *oto.theclinics.com*

airway obstruction in children. There are a number of reasons why even a small amount of inflammation in the subglottis can result in airway compromise:

The subglottis is the only region of the airway bounded by a complete cartilaginous ring that prevents the airway's outward expansion in the face of edema.
The pseudostratified, ciliated, columnar respiratory epithelium lining the subglottis is loosely adherent to the underlying perichondrium.
Numerous mucus-secreting glands lie within the subgottis mucosa.

Even 1 mm of edema in the normal pediatric subglottis reduces its area by more than 50%.

Croup is typically caused by respiratory viruses, with parainfluenza I, II, and III accounting for up to 80% of cases. Parainfluenza I is the etiologic agent in 50% to 70% of patients who are hospitalized for croup [2]. Other pathogens implicated in the pathogenesis of croup include adenovirus, respiratory syncytial virus, varicella, herpes simplex virus measles, enteroviruses, *Mycoplasma pneumoniae*, and influenza viruses A and B [3,4]. Influenza-mediated croup is associated with a more severe disease course compared with parainfluenza [5]. The virus is transmitted through inhalation and infects the epithelial cells of the laryngeal and tracheal mucosa, causing edema and glandular hypersecretion. Bacteria are an infrequent cause of croup, although bacterial tracheitis, which can result in significant airway obstruction and even death from the accumulation of pseudomembranes and fibrinous exudate within the airway, is most often caused by *Staphylococcus aureus* and *Streptococcus pyogenes*. Fungi and mycobacteria are extremely rare infectious causes of laryngotracheobronchitis and, when noted, should raise suspicion of an underlying immunodeficiency.

Noninfectious narrowing of the subglottis caused by congenital stenosis, internal or external laryngeal trauma, thermal injury, mass lesions such as hemangioma, and aspirated foreign bodies may present with clinical and radiographic findings similar to acute infectious laryngotracheobronchitis. Intubation may result in a series of changes within the subglottis (beginning with inflammatory edema and perichondritis) that occasionally progresses to mature subglottic stenosis. During the evolution of subglottic stenosis, the patient may present with symptoms that are not differentiable from viral croup. The role of supraesophageal reflux in the pathogenesis of croup remains unclear. A study by Contencin and Narcy [6] demonstrated that 100% of eight patients who had recurrent croup had pH probe studies consistent with reflux.

Epidemiology

Croup is the most common cause of stridor in children and accounts for up to 15% of emergency department and primary care visits for respiratory infections in the United States [2]. It most commonly affects children, with its peak incidence at age 2 years; however, there are isolated reports of cases in adults [7–9]. The annual incidence ranges from 1.5% to 6% in children younger than 6 years [7]. There is a slight male preponderance (male-to-female ratio, 3:2) [7]. The incidence of croup is highest in the fall and early winter months.

Most cases of croup are managed in the primary care or emergency room setting, with 1.5% to 31% of patients requiring admission [10] and less than 5% requiring endotracheal intubation [11]. The mortality from croup has greatly decreased over the past 50 years secondary to advances in pediatric intensive care and airway management. Nevertheless, there are still isolated reports of mortality from croup, emphasizing the need for vigilant observation and early airway intervention in severe cases [12].

Clinical presentation

The patient who has croup typically presents with a hoarse voice, a "barking" cough, a low-grade fever, and variable degrees of stridor and respiratory distress. In contrast to epiglottitis, children who have croup typically present with a viral prodrome that may include rhinorrhea, cough, and sore throat for 1 to 2 days before the onset of the classic croup symptoms. A risk factor evaluation should always be sought, with careful attention paid to the patient's neonatal and intubation history.

Examination findings may be similar to those of a viral upper respiratory tract infection, but children who have croup typically do not present with the toxic appearance characteristic of epiglottitis. A low-grade fever is often noted on examination, as is the finding of a hoarse voice, the characteristic high-pitched barking cough, and stridor. An evaluation for signs of respiratory distress including tachypnea, retractions, nasal flaring, agitation, lethargy, oxygen desaturation, and cyanosis should be performed. The Westley score is a tool used in various institutions to characterize the severity of respiratory distress in children who have croup (Table 1) [13]. The clinical efficacy of this and other scoring systems has not been extensively evaluated, and their utility remains controversial. The complete examination of the patient who has croup should include an evaluation for the presence of cutaneous hemangiomas, which may raise the possibility of a subglottic hemangioma, especially if present in a patient younger than 6 months who has croup.

Croup usually presents in children between age 6 months and 3 years, with a discrete episode of symptoms lasting between 3 and 7 days. Up to 5% of children may have more than one episode [14]. Patients who are younger than 6 months when they first present with croup, those who have an unusually long duration of symptoms (> 1 week), those who have unusually severe symptoms, and those who have recurrent croup should be evaluated for congenital or acquired airway narrowing.

Spasmodic croup is a nebulous condition that presents with a history and physical examination similar to viral croup without the associated infectious clinical findings. The patient is usually acutely symptomatic at night, with

Table 1
Westley croup scoring system

Indicator of disease severity	Score
Stridor	
None	0
Only with agitation/excitement	1
At rest with stethoscope	2
At rest without stethoscope	3
Retraction	
None	0
Mild	1
Moderate	2
Severe	3
Air entry	
Normal	0
Decreased	1
Severely decreased	2
Cyanosis	
None	0
With agitation	4
At rest	5
Level of consciousness	
Normal	0
Altered mental status	5

Mild respiratory distress = score <3; moderate respiratory distress = score 3–6; severe respiratory distress = score >6.

rapid resolution of the condition occurring over a period of 24 to 48 hours [12]. The etiology of spasmodic croup is unknown but may be allergic. The differential diagnosis of croup is listed in Box 1.

Diagnosis and initial management

The diagnosis of croup should be made clinically. The characteristic barking cough, hoarse voice, stridor, and low-grade fever in the absence of the previously mentioned risk factors may obviate the need for additional diagnostic tests, which are nonspecific. If the patient presents with significant respiratory distress, expeditious coordinated care should be arranged between the otolaryngologist, anesthesiologist, and critical care intensivist. Measures to secure the airway are of utmost priority. Supplemental humidified oxygen and racemic epinephrine may be administered until definitive intervention to secure the airway can be undertaken. Care must be taken during this period to avoid excessive stimulation of the child because this may exacerbate the airway compromise.

If the patient is stable and the diagnosis is in question, high-kilovoltage plain films of the airway and a chest radiograph may be obtained to rule out findings suggestive of another etiology. Anteroposterior films may demonstrate symmetric subglottic narrowing ("steeple sign"), although this may

---

Box 1. Differential diagnosis of croup

Congenital
Laryngomalacia
Vocal cord paralysis
Laryngeal web
Subglottic stenosis
Subglottic hemangioma
Tracheomalacia

Infectious/inflammatory
Respiratory papillomatosis
Epiglottitis
Peritonsillar abscess
Deep neck space infection
Diphtheria
Bacterial tracheitis
Mycobacteria
Laryngeal candidiasis
Angioedema
Wegener's granulomatosis
Extraesophageal reflux

Traumatic/toxic
Acquired subglottic stenosis
Inhalational injury
Foreign body

Vascular
Innominate artery compression
Double aortic arch
Aberrant subclavian artery
Pulmonary artery sling

Neoplastic

---

be absent in up to 50% of cases and may be present in the absence of croup (Fig. 1) [14]. Flexible fiberoptic laryngoscopy has a limited ability to evaluate the subglottis but may be sought to rule out pathology of the supraglottis and vocal cords when the diagnosis is unclear. Direct microlaryngoscopy and bronchoscopy (MLB) is the gold standard for the diagnosis of airway lesions and should be employed (1) when the diagnosis of croup is in question after noninvasive testing, (2) in the evaluation of a patient who has atypical croup, (3) when bacterial tracheitis is suspected, and (4) in patients who have risk factors suggestive of underlying airway pathologies. If possible, the patient

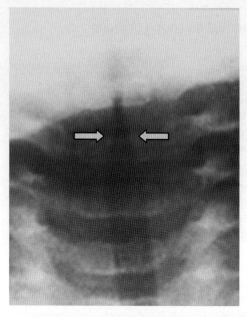

Fig. 1. Anteroposterior neck film demonstrating steeple sign (*arrows*).

should be at his or her baseline before performing MLB to most accurately assess the airway in the absence of acute edema. Moreover, MLB of the acutely infected airway may result in exacerbation of the edema secondary to manipulation, which may worsen the patient's airway obstruction.

Definitive management

When the airway is deemed stable and the diagnosis of croup is established, supportive and medical measures should be employed in the primary care or emergency room setting. Sixty percent of children present with mild croup symptoms and are often discharged from the emergency department without any treatment [15]. Supportive measures may include placing the patient in a cool-mist "croup" tent; medical options include possible administration of oxygen, racemic epinephrine, and systemic steroids. The value of cool mist, which was the mainstay of therapy for croup for over a century, is controversial. Cool mist is thought to improve airflow through the edematous subglottis by decreasing the viscosity of secretions. A recent meta-analysis and randomized controlled trial failed to demonstrate the benefit of cool mist in the outcome of moderate and severe croup [16,17].

Due to their significant anti-inflammatory effects, systemic steroids are the mainstay of therapy for patients with croup and can be administered by way of nebulization and oral or intravenous routes. The liberal administration of steroids for mild to severe croup significantly reduces the severity and duration of croup episodes and is thought to be responsible for the dramatic decrease in the need for hospital or intensive care admissions and endotracheal intubation [18]. In a double-blinded controlled trial, Bjornson and colleagues [15] reported a statistically significant reduction in symptoms, parental stress, and the need for subsequent care after administration of a single dose of oral dexamethasone (0.6 mg/kg) to patients who had mild croup. Two recent randomized trials demonstrated similar efficacy of low-dose (0.15 mg/kg) and high-dose (0.6 mg/kg) dexamethasone in reducing croup symptoms [19,20]. Amir and colleagues [21] recently demonstrated no difference in the outcome of mild to moderate croup after administration of oral or intramuscular steroids. Donaldson and colleagues [22] noted similar findings in their study assessing intramuscular versus oral steroids in patients who had moderate to severe croup. Both of these studies highlight the utility of orai steroid therapy due to ease of administration in the ambulatory setting. The role of continued steroid therapy after the initial dose is unclear, but it may be considered for patients who require hospital admission for treatment.

Adrenergic agents are highly effective at reducing airway edema by rapidly constricting mucosal blood vessels and reducing vascular permeability [12]. Due to the potential for side effects including agitation, tachycardia, and hypertension, the use of nebulized (racemic or levo-) epinephrine is commonly reserved for patients who have moderate to severe respiratory distress. The rapid onset of action of epinephrine (10–30 minutes) makes its use beneficial in these severe cases because the anti-inflammatory effects of steroids may not be appreciated for several hours after administration. A recent randomized controlled trial assessing the efficacy of levo-epinephrine in combination with systemic or inhaled steroids demonstrated significant improvement in the outcome of patients who had moderate and severe croup when treated with combination therapy [23]. Patients treated with epinephrine need to be observed for at least 3 to 4 hours after administration due to the possibility of symptom regression after the initial beneficial effects subside.

Heliox is a low-density alternative to oxygen that is thought to improve gas flow through the compromised airway. The value of heliox in the treatment of croup has recently been assessed. In a randomized controlled trial of 29 patients, Weber and colleagues [24] reported similar benefits from the use of heliox and racemic epinephrine.

Admission to the medical ward or ICU should be considered (1) if the patient has evidence of continued respiratory distress after initial therapy, (2) if the patient presents with severe croup, or (3) if the social situation does not permit easy access to medical care in case of worsening symptomatology. Hospital care is largely supportive, although further medical management and rarely intubation are occasionally necessary. Otolaryngology consultation should be sought when

Significant airway compromise is present
Diagnosis of croup is in question

Patient has recurrent or prolonged croup
Suspicion of bacterial tracheitis is present
Congenital or acquired airway pathology is diagnosed

Intubation should be reserved for cases of severe croup refractory to medical measures. Care must be taken to use the smallest possible endotracheal tube to avoid traumatizing the inflamed mucosa. The patient may be extubated after detection of an air leak.

Surgical management for croup is limited to MLB, as previously indicated. Tracheotomy is rarely required to secure the airway. A discussion of the surgical management of predisposing airway pathologies is beyond the scope of this article.

Summary

Over the past century, advances in the management of croup have transformed this condition from an almost certain death sentence to a relatively benign self-limited condition. A careful history and physical examination are critical to the diagnosis of croup and essential to ruling out less common conditions that mimic or presdispose to acute viral laryngotracheobronchitis. As with any airway condition, the first consideration in a patient who has croup should be rapid airway assessment and stabilization. When this step is complete, croup is almost always manageable with supportive and medical measures in the primary care or emergency room setting, with surgery reserved for diagnosis and management of complications.

Epiglottitis

Epiglottitis is an acute inflammation of the epiglottis or supraglottis that may lead to the rapid onset of life-threatening airway obstruction and is considered an otolaryngologic emergency. Since the widespread implementation of a conjugate vaccine for *Haemophilus influenzae* type b (Hib) nearly 2 decades ago, the incidence of epiglottitis has significantly declined in children. Securing the airway should be accomplished immediately in a controlled setting. Coordinated communication between the otolaryngologist, anesthesiologist, and intensivist is vital to the care provided to these critically ill patients.

Historical accounts of George Washington's death suggest that he succumbed to acute epiglottitis. One early December morning in 1799, George Washington awoke with a severe sore throat. Throughout the day, his condition rapidly deteriorated as he developed difficulty in swallowing, an unintelligibly muffled voice, and persistent restlessness. Although a tracheotomy was suggested by one physician in attendance at his bedside, the procedure was not well-practiced at that time, and a series of bloodlettings were performed instead. He expired less than 24 hours from the onset of his symptoms [25].

Pathogenesis

The epiglottis comprises a leaf-shaped elastic cartilage with overlying loose connective tissue and a thin epithelial layer. It arises from the posterior tongue base and covers the laryngeal inlet during swallowing. Any inflammation of the epiglottis can easily spread to the attached aryepiglottic folds and the arytenoid soft tissues, causing a more generalized supraglottitis. Bacterial invasion of the mucosa leads to fulminant infection, with rapid evolution of edema causing severe, life-threatening obstruction of the upper airway (Fig. 2).

Traditionally, epiglottitis was most commonly caused by Hib and primarily reported in children aged 2 to 7 years. The introduction of the Hib conjugate vaccine in 1988 dramatically changed the epidemiology of acute epiglottitis. The Hib vaccine is recommended at age 2 months, 4 months, 6 months (depending on the brand), and 12 to 15 months. By 1996, the incidence of invasive Hib disease among children younger than 5 years declined by more than 99% [26]. Today supraglottitis is diagnosed more often in adults, and a variety of causative pathogens have been identified [27].

No single organism is considered the principal cause of epiglottitis. Despite the dramatic decrease of Hib-related infections after introduction of the vaccine, recent reports have shown that Hib may still cause epiglottitis despite adequate vaccination [28,29]. It should be noted, however, that vaccination failure may have prevailed with use of the older, purified polysaccharide vaccine [28]. Infectious agents in the postvaccination era associated with epiglottitis include group A *Streptococcus pneumoniae, Staphylococcus aureus, Klebsiella pneumoniae, Haemophilus parainfluenzae,* and beta-hemolytic streptococci (group A, B, C, and F) [27,30–32]. Candidal and viral infections (herpes simplex type 1, varicella-zoster, and parainfluenza) have also been implicated, particularly in immunocompromised individuals [33–35].

Noninfectious causes such as direct trauma and thermal injury may also lead to swelling of the epiglottis [36]. Injury to the epiglottis secondary to ingestion of hot foods or liquids, caustic agents, foreign bodies, smoke

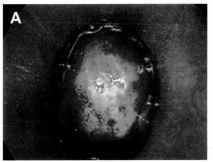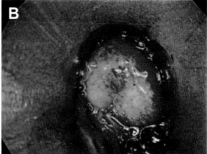

Fig. 2. Acute epiglottitis with views of the cherry red epiglottis on direct laryngoscopy. (*Courtesy of* M. Bitner, MD, Atlanta, GA).

inhalation, angioedema, and sidestream exposure to "crack" cocaine have been reported in children and adults. The aforementioned clinical entities often present with symptoms and radiographic findings similar to acute infectious epiglottitis, including fever, sore throat, dysphagia, drooling, leukocytosis, and the "thumb sign" on lateral neck film. It is not uncommon to encounter these circumstances in mentally afflicted patients or individuals who have communication disorders, and therefore, a thorough history and evaluation of the aerodigestive tract is essential when a noninfectious source is suspected [36–39].

Epidemiology

At the Children's Hospital of Buffalo, a rate of 3.5 cases of epiglottitis per 10,000 admissions in 1969 to 1977 decreased to 0.3 cases per 10,000 admissions in 1995 to 2003. Hib was the causative organism identified in 84% of the cases in the earlier years, but was completely absent in the later segment of the study [30]. A 5-year retrospective review of the incidence of epiglottitis at the Children's Hospital of Philadelphia indicated a frequency of 10.9 per 10,000 admissions before 1990. Only 1.8 episodes per 10,000 admissions were noted 5 years after introduction of the vaccine [32].

A Finland study also demonstrated a decreased incidence from a prevaccination era incidence of 50 and 60 cases annually in 1985 and 1986, respectively, to only 2 cases in 1992 after widespread administration of the Hib vaccine [40]. In a Swedish study, the incidence of epiglottitis also decreased substantially from 20.9 in 1987 to 0.9 in 1996 for children younger than 5 years [41].

The annual incidence of acute epiglottitis in adults has risen significantly in Israel from a rate of 0.88 (1986–1990) to 2.1 (1991–1995) to 3.1 (1996–2000) [27]. A comparison of cases between adults and children in Australia revealed a significant difference in the postvaccine era (84% versus 17%, respectively) [42].

There is a male preponderance of acute epiglottitis, with male-to-female ratios ranging from 1.2:1 to 4:1 [27,35,43,44]. Most studies have not demonstrated a seasonal variation in the incidence of acute epiglottitis [27,35,45]. Mortality rates have decreased considerably since the introduction of the Hib vaccine and the consequent shift in disease from young children to adults. Death rates are now less than 1% for children but approach 7% for adults. When deaths have occurred, a large percentage transpired due to delay in diagnosis or shortly after arrival at a medical facility for appropriate care [35,44].

Clinical presentation

Epiglottitis typically presents with acute onset of sore throat and fever. Rapid progression to difficulty swallowing, drooling, restlessness, and stridor or air hunger ensues [27,35,43,44]. The clinical triad of the "three Ds" (drooling, dysphagia, and distress) is a classic presentation. A viral pro-drome and cough are seldom observed with acute epiglottitis and are more often witnessed in association with croup.

Patients generally appear toxic and anxious. Often they assume the "sniff-ing position," with the head hyperextended and nose pointed superiorly in an effort to maintain a patent airway. Vocalization is quite painful, and the patient may speak with a "hot potato" or muffled voice. The laryngotracheal complex is usually exquisitely tender to palpation, especially in the region of the hyoid bone. This finding alone undeniably raises suspicion for the diagno-sis of epiglottitis [44,46]. Nonspecific lymphadenopathy may also be present.

Diagnosis and initial management

When epiglottitis is suspected, immediate coordinated care should be ar-ranged between otolaryngology, anesthesiology, and critical care intensivists. Measures to secure the airway are of utmost priority. Supplemental humid-ified oxygen and racemic epinephrine may be administered until definitive intervention to secure the airway can be undertaken.

Factors characteristically associated with airway obstruction include intolerance of secretions, diabetes mellitus, rapid onset of symptoms, and presence of epiglottic abscess [27,35,45,47,48]. In the Rhode Island experi-ence, 68% of children and 21% of adults required airway intervention as part of their management [35]. Smaller percentages have been reported in other studies that have reviewed primarily adult outcomes [43,45].

In patients who have mild to moderate respiratory distress or in older, cooperative patients, the classic cherry red epiglottis may be visualized with gentle compression of the anterior tongue with a tongue depressor (see Fig. 2). Indirect visualization of the larynx with flexible laryngoscopy may also be used to confirm the diagnosis [27]. Although no reports exist to document that these maneuvers are unsafe, there has always been concern for provoking anxiety and triggering or exacerbating respiratory distress with these stimulating methods.

The patient should be expeditiously transported to the operating room to secure the airway. All emergency airway equipment, including oral airways, laryngeal mask anesthesia, laryngoscopes, rigid bronchoscopes, flexible intubating bronchoscopes, jet ventilation ports, and instruments for crico-thyrotomy/tracheotomy should be readily available by the time the patient arrives in the operating suite. Mask ventilation with orotracheal intubation is attempted before any other actions are taken. If intubation is not possible, a surgical airway with cricothyrotomy or tracheotomy is performed.

It is recommended that all other diagnostic tests (laboratory, imaging, and so forth) and placement of intravenous lines be postponed until the airway is secure. In older children and adults who do not have respiratory distress and who have at least a 50% laryngeal lumen on flexible laryngoscopy, it is reasonable to forgo intubation and monitor the patient closely. It should be noted, however, that with this practice, rapid respiratory compromise may develop in a delayed manner, necessitating emergent airway intervention [27,35,49]. All patients who have epiglottitis should be admitted to the ICU for observation and definitive treatment. Supplies for immediate endotracheal intubation or emergency tracheotomy should be available at the bedside for patients who do not have a secured airway.

A complete blood cell count with differential, blood cultures, and epiglottic cultures (when an artificial airway has been placed) are obtained after the airway is secure and the patient is stable. Elevated white blood cell counts are frequently present, but positive blood culture results are extremely variable (6%–15%) [27,35,42,43].

Lateral neck radiographs may demonstrate the classic thumb sign, indicative of the severe edema involving the epiglottis (Fig. 3). The poor sensitivity (38%) and specificity (78%) of plain films limits the utility of this radiographic modality in the current age of technologic advances, whereby the larynx can be safely and accurately visualized with flexible laryngoscopy [50]. Contrasted CT scan of the neck may also indicate the presence of epiglottic edema and possibly phlegmon or abscess in the epiglottis or the base of tongue. The incidence of epiglottic abscesses appears to be increasing concomitantly with the rise in acute epiglottitis in adults. Patients who have epiglottic abscesses typically have a more severe course of the disease and a higher incidence of airway obstruction [27,51].

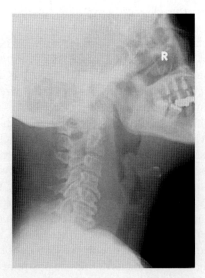

Fig. 3. Lateral neck film demonstrating thumb sign with edema of the epiglottis. (*Courtesy of* M. Bitner, MD, Atlanta, GA).

Definitive management

Securing the airway is the initial step in the management of epiglottitis. Broad-spectrum antibiotic coverage, typically a second- or third-generation cephalosporin (eg, cefuroxime or amoxicillin and potassium clavulanate), is directed to cover staphylococcus and streptococcus organisms for 7 to 10 days. Steroids are commonly employed to decrease mucosal edema of the epiglottis, but no data exist in the literature to prove any benefit from their use (Fig. 4) [35,51–55].

Abscess of the epiglottis is treated by incision and drainage. If the abscess is present and identified at admission, it is addressed at the time of airway intervention. Air leak tests around the endotracheal tube and direct

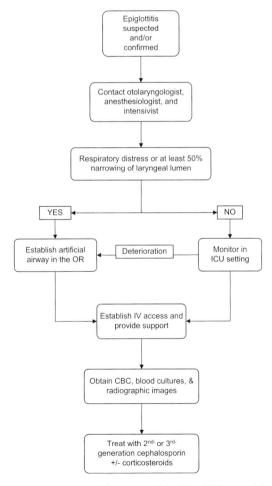

Fig. 4. Emergency treatment protocol for acute epiglottitis. CBC, complete blood count; IV, intravenous; OR, operating room.

visualization of the larynx after 24 to 48 hours of therapy facilitate decisions concerning the timing of extubation.

Summary

The dramatic decrease in the incidence of acute epiglottitis in the postvaccine era necessitates a high index of suspicion in patients presenting with the rapid onset of signs and symptoms consistent with epiglottitis. Because this entity has shifted from children to adults, a more conservative approach with close ICU monitoring is advocated in a select group of patients. With established protocols to provide rapid treatment and to secure the airway, excellent outcomes are expected to continue for most patients.

References

[1] Baskett TF. Joseph O'Dwyer and laryngeal intubation. Resuscitation 2007;74:211–4.
[2] Molodow RE, Defendi GL, Muniz A. Croup. In: A Meyers, editor. Emedicine textbook of pediatrics. Available at: http://www.emedicine.com. August, 2006.
[3] Myer CM. Inflammatory diseases of the pediatric airway. In: Cotton RT, Myers CM, editors. Practical pediatric otolaryngology. Philadelphia: Lippincott-Raven; 1999. p. 547–59.
[4] Baugh R, Gilmore BB. Infectious croup: a critical review. Otolaryngol Head Neck Surg 1986;95:40–6.
[5] Peltola V, Heikkinen T, Ruuskanen O. Clinical courses of croup caused by influenza and parainfluenza viruses. Pediatr Infect Dis J 2002;21:76–8.
[6] Contencin PH, Narcy P. Gastropharyngeal reflux in infants and children. A pharyngeal pH monitoring study. Arch Otolaryngol Head Neck Surg 1992;118:1028–30.
[7] Denny FW, Murphy TF, Clyde WA, et al. Croup: an 11-year study in pediatric practice. Pediatrics 1983;71:871–6.
[8] Woo PC, Young K, Tsang KW, et al. Adult croup: a rare but more severe condition. Respiration 2000;67:684–8.
[9] Nakamaya JM, Tokeshai J. A case report of adult croup: a new old problem. Hawaii Med J 2005;64:246–7.
[10] Marx A, Torok TJ, Holman MJ, et al. Pediatric hospitalizations for croup (laryngotracheitis): biennial increases associated with human parainfluenza virus 1 epidemics. J Infect Dis 1997;176:1423–7.
[11] Wagener JS, Landau LI, Olinsky PD. Management of children hospitalized for laryngotracheobronchitis. Pediatr Pulmonol 1986;2:159–62.
[12] Fitzgerald DA. The assessment and management of croup. Paediatr Respir Rev 2006;7: 73–81.
[13] Westley CR, Cotton EK, Brooks JG. Nebulized racemic epinephrine by IPPB for the treatment of croup: a double-blind study. Am J Dis Child 1978;132:484–7.
[14] Stroud RH, Friedman NR. An update on inflammatory disorders of the pediatric airway: epiglottitis, croup, and tracheitis. Am J Otolaryngol 2001;22:268–75.
[15] Bjornson CL, Klassen TP, Williamson J, et al. A randomized trial of a single dose of oral dexamethasone for mild croup. N Engl J Med 2004;351:1306–13.
[16] Moore M, Little P. Humidified air inhalation for treating croup: a systematic review and meta-analysis. Fam Pract 2007;24(4):295–301.
[17] Scolnik D, Coates AL, Stephens D, et al. Controlled delivery of high vs low humidity vs mist therapy for croup in emergency departments: a randomized controlled trial. JAMA 2006; 295:1274–80.

[18] Fitzgerald DA, Kilham HA. Croup: assessment and evidence-based management. Med J Aust 2003;179:372–7.

[19] Fifoot AA, Ting JY. Comparison between single-dose oral prednisolone and oral dexamethasone in the treatment of croup: a randomized, double blinded clinical trial. Emerg Med Australas 2007;19:51–8.

[20] Chub-Upparkarn S, Sangsupawanich P. A randomized comparison of dexamethasone 0.15mg/kg versus 0.6mg/kg for the treatment of moderate to severe croup. Int J Pediatr Otorhinolaryngol 2007;71:473–7.

[21] Amir L, Hubermann H, Halevi A, et al. Oral betamethasone versus intramuscular dexamethasone for the treatment of mild to moderate viral croup: a prospective randomized trial. Pediatr Emerg Care 2006;22:541–4.

[22] Donaldson D, Poleski D, Knipple E, et al. Intramuscular versus oral dexamethasone for the treatment of moderate to severe croup: a randomized, double-blind trial. Acad Emerg Med 2003;10:16–21.

[23] Duman M, Ozdemir D, Atasever S. Nebulised L-epinephrine and steroid combination in the treatment of moderate to severe croup. Clin Drug Investig 2005;25:183–9.

[24] Weber JE, Chudnofsky CR, Younger JG, et al. A randomized comparison of helium-oxygen mixture (heliox) and racemic adrenaline for the treatment of moderate to severe croup. Pediatrics 2001;107:e96.

[25] Morens DM. Death of a president. N Engl J Med 1999;341(24):1845–9.

[26] CDC. Progress toward elimination of Haemophilus influenzae type b invasive disease among infants and children—United States, 1998–2000. MMWR Morb Mortal Wkly Rep 2002;51: 234–7.

[27] Berger G, Landau T, Berger S. The rising incidence of adult acute epiglottitis and epiglottic abscess. Am J Otolaryngol 2003;24:374–83.

[28] Gonzalez Valdepena H, Wald ER, Rose E, et al. Epiglottitis and Haemophilus influenzae immunization: the Pittsburgh experience—a five-year review. Pediatrics 1995;96:424–7.

[29] Tanner K, Fitzsimmons G, Carrol ED, et al. Lesson of the week: Haemophilus influenzae type b epiglottitis as a cause of acute upper airways obstruction in children. BMJ 2002; 325:1099–100.

[30] Faden H. The dramatic change in the epidemiology of pediatric epiglottitis. Pediatr Emerg Care 2006;22:443–4.

[31] Isaacson G, Isaacson DM. Pediatric epiglottitis caused by group G beta-hemolytic Streptococcus. Pediatr Infect Dis J 2003;22:846–7.

[32] Gorelick MH, Baker MD. Epiglottitis in children, 1979 through 1992. Effects of Haemophilus influenzae type b immunization. Arch Pediatr Adolesc Med 1994;148:47–50.

[33] Cole S, Zawin M, Lundberg B, et al. Candida epiglottitis in an adult with acute nonlymphocytic leukemia. Am J Med 1987;82:662–4.

[34] Walsh TJ, Gray WC. Candida epiglottitis in immunocompromised patients. Chest 1987;91: 482–5.

[35] Mayo-Smith MF, Spinale JW, Donskey CJ, et al. Acute epiglottitis: an 18-year experience in Rhode Island. Chest 1995;108:1640–7.

[36] Kornak JM, Freije JE, Campbell BH. Caustic and thermal epiglottitis in the adult. Otolaryngol Head Neck Surg 1996;114:310–2.

[37] Kharasch S, Vinci R, Reece R. Esophagitis, epiglottitis, and cocaine alkaloid ("crack"): "accidental" poisoning or child abuse? Pediatrics 1990;86:117–9.

[38] Sataloff RT. Upper airway distress and crack cocaine use [letter]. Otolaryngol Head Neck Surg 1994;111:115.

[39] Savitt DL, Colagiovanni S. Crack cocaine-related epiglottitis [letter]. Ann Emerg Med 1991; 20:322–3.

[40] Takala AK, Peltola H, Eskola J. Disappearance of epiglottitis during large-scale vaccination with Haemophilus influenzae type B conjugate vaccine among children in Finland. Laryngoscope 1994;104:731–5.

[41] Garpenholt O, Hugosson S, Fredlund H, et al. Epiglottitis in Sweden before and after introduction of vaccination against *Haemophilus influenzae* type b. Pediatr Infect Dis J 1999;18:
490–3.

[42] Wood N, Menzies R, McIntyre P. Epiglottitis in Sydney before and after the introduction of vaccination against *Haemophilus influenzae* type b disease. Intern Med J 2005;
35:530–5.

[43] Price IM, Preyra I, Fernandes CM, et al. Adult epiglottitis: a five-year retrospective chart
review in a major urban centre. CJEM 2005;7:387–90.

[44] Carey MJ. Epiglottitis in adults. Am J Emerg Med 1996;14:421–4.

[45] Katori H, Tsukuda M. Acute epiglottitis: analysis of factors associated with airway intervention. J Laryngol Otol 2005;119:967–72.

[46] Ehara H. Tenderness over the hyoid bone can indicate epiglottitis in adults. J Am Board Fam
Med 2006;19:517–20.

[47] Solomon P, Weisbrod M, Irish JC, et al. Adult epiglottitis: the Toronto Hospital experience.
J Otolaryngol 1998;27:332–6.

[48] Deeb ZE, Yenson AC, DeFries HO. Acute epiglottitis in the adult. Laryngoscope 1985;95:
289–91.

[49] Gerrish SP, Jones AS, Watson DM, et al. Adult epiglottitis. BMJ 1987;295:1183–4.

[50] Stankiewicz JA, Bowes AK. Croup and epiglottitis: a radiologic study. Laryngoscope 1985;
95:1159–60.

[51] Wolf M, Strauss B, Kronenberg J, et al. Conservative management of adult epiglottitis.
Laryngoscope 1990;100:183–5.

[52] Hebert PC, Ducic Y, Boisvert D, et al. Adult epiglottitis in a Canadian setting. Laryngoscope
1998;108:64–9.

[53] Murrage KJ, Janzen VD, Ruby RR. Epiglottitis: adult and pediatric comparisons. J Otolaryngol 1988;17:194–8.

[54] Dort JC, Frohlich AM, Tate RB. Acute epiglottitis in adults: diagnosis and treatment in
43 patients. J Otolaryngol 1994;23:281–5.

[55] Frantz TD, Rasgon BM, Quesenbery CP Jr. Acute epiglottitis in adults. Analysis of
129 cases. JAMA 1994;272:1358–60.

ELSEVIER
SAUNDERS

Otolaryngol Clin N Am
41 (2008) 567–580

OTOLARYNGOLOGIC
CLINICS
OF NORTH AMERICA

The Difficult Airway

Benjamin D. Liess, MD, Troy D. Scheidt, MD,
Jerry W. Templer, MD*

*Department of Otolaryngology Head and Neck Surgery, University of
Missouri–Columbia School of Medicine, One Hospital Drive, Columbia, MO 65212, USA*

Encountering a patient with a tenuous upper airway is a daunting situation for most physicians. The fate of the patient depends on prepared professionals trained in the evaluation and management of the airway. While some causes of airway obstruction are evident, many difficult airway situations manifest at induction of anesthesia. Unanticipated difficulty encountered during routine attempted intubation may quickly deteriorate into a life-threatening emergency if ill prepared. The degree of difficulty is often influenced by the patient's anatomy and health status, the clinical setting, and the ability of the practitioner [1]. Otolaryngologists and anesthesiologists should jointly plan the management of the difficult airway to ensure successful control.

No universally accepted definition of the difficult airway exists, but in broad terms, difficult airway control may be defined as problematic ventilation using a face mask, incomplete laryngoscopic visualization, or as a difficult intubation with standard airway equipment. Difficult ventilation is the inability to deliver the necessary tidal volume via the face mask even when using an oral or nasal airway and necessitating another device such as the laryngeal mask airway. Difficult laryngoscopy is impaired visualization of the true vocal cords despite elaborate external laryngeal repositioning, more specifically a Cormack and Lehane grade 3 or 4 (Box 1) [2]. Difficult intubation has been defined as requiring external laryngeal manipulation, difficult laryngoscopy requiring greater than three attempts at intubation, intubation requiring nonstandard equipment or approaches, or the inability to intubate using all available methods.

Establishment of standards of care, a management algorithm, and a working knowledge of common equipment are crucial. Organization and coordination among otolaryngologists, anesthesiologists, emergency

---

* Corresponding author.
E-mail address: templerj@health.missouri.edu (J.W. Templer).

0030-6665/08/$ - see front matter © 2008 Elsevier Inc. All rights reserved.
doi:10.1016/j.otc.2008.01.007

Box 1. Cormack Lehane scale [2]

Visualization of the glottis during direct laryngoscopy
  with Macintosh blade
1. Full view of the glottis
2. Partial vocal fold or posterior commissure view
3. Epiglottic tip visualized
4. No exposure of glottic structures

---

room physicians, and hospital staff are critical to foster a working environment that has a positive impact on patient outcome. Recognizing deficits and developing a systematic approach to the airway is an important step for improving patient safety and providing good outcomes.

Complications related to management of the difficult airway have significant impact on our patients. The inability to obtain and maintain an airway after induction with general anesthesia is a cause of nearly one third of anesthesia complications, with a large portion of these resulting in significant morbidity or mortality [3,4]. The incidence of difficult intubation in the operating room ranges between 1.15% and 3.80% [5], with failed attempts in 0.05% to 0.35% of cases [6,7]. In the emergency department, difficult intubation occurs in 3.0% to 5.3% [6,7] of cases with failure rates ranging from 0.5% to 1.1% [6,7]. Hypoxia from the difficult airway is commonly due to [8]:

1. Excessive number of attempts performed by different operators unsuccessfully
2. Subsequent attempts with the same devices
3. Inadequate oxygenation between attempts
4. Aspiration of gastric contents during face mask ventilation
5. Traumatic edema of the laryngeal auditus

Evaluation

Patient evaluation may occur in a controlled setting in the clinic or preoperative holding area or while the patient is decompensating in the emergency room, operating room, or out in the field. Both the environment and patient stability dictate the scope of evaluation and management. The ability to quickly assess a situation, plan the approach, and intervene by successfully securing an airway is vital. A breadth of understanding of the airway anatomy in relation to patient age and underlying etiology are key to prepare for the subsequent intervention.

Elective

If the situation is not urgent, a detailed history is obtained. The progression or regression and severity of symptoms should be noted. The history must also address difficulty with previous general anesthesia, sleep apnea or snoring, head and neck abnormalities, and other coexisting disease that might impair the airway or prevent standard intubation.

Adults

Adults with an impaired airway may present with a myriad of symptoms secondary to the underlying etiology. Signs and symptoms include dyspnea at rest or on exertion, stridor, neck swelling, voice changes, hemoptysis, dysphagia, odynophagia, and cough. Causes of airway impingement vary greatly and include such categories as infection, malignancy, and trauma (Table 1).

In an adult, the examination should carefully note facial and neck masses and deformities, scars, quality of dentition, maxillary and mandibular position, pharyngeal structures, and neck mobility. Flexible fiber-optic endoscopy provides a "tour" of the interior of the nose, nasopharynx, pharynx, larynx, and upper trachea. This endoscopy is the most important factor in determining the status of the upper airway and the cause of the impairment.

Predictors of a significantly difficult or impossible intubation in adults include the following [8–13]:

1. Interincisor distance 3 cm or less
2. Thyro-mental distance 6 cm or less
3. Maxillary dentition interfering with jaw thrust
4. Malampati classification 4 (Box 2)
5. Neck in fixed flexion
6. Extreme head and neck radiation changes, scarring, or large masses

Additionally, some authors suggest increased age, male sex, history of obstructive sleep apnea, high body mass index, and pretracheal soft tissue may portend a challenging issue [14–16]. However, other authors did not find high body mass index, neck mobility, increased age, thyromental distance, male sex, or high Malampati score as reliable measures in predicting a difficult airway [15–18]. Additional factors that may affect a practitioner's ability to manage the airway include amount of facial hair, dentition, and a history of chronic obstructive pulmonary disease, asthma, or snoring [19].

Children

Parents of young children are questioned about noisy breathing during exercise, at rest or when feeding, previous surgeries or intubations, neck pain, fever, recent upper respiratory infections, birth trauma, and congenital anomalies. The history of an unexplained coughing episode is suggestive of a foreign body of the larynx, trachea, or bronchi.

The physical examination must note the respiratory rate, nasal flaring, and accessory muscle use. Stridor, cough, and voice changes are frequently seen. Generally, most cases of acute airway compromise in children are due to infections, foreign bodies, and trauma; however, congenital malformations, neoplasia, and iatrogenic injury are additional considerations.

Table 1
Differential diagnosis of airway impairment

	(K)Congenital	Infectious	Toxins and trauma	Tumor	Endocrine	Neurologic	Systemic
Above the larynx	Congenital syndromes (Pierre Robin, Treacher Collins, mucopolysaccharidoses, Down's) tonsil and adenoid hypertrophy, micrognathia, nasal turbinate hypertrophy, lingual thyroid, choanal atresia, macroglossia, nasoseptal deformity	Submandibular, peritonsillar, retropharyngeal, parapharyngeal abscesses, mononucleosis, diphtheria, Ludwig's angina	Maxillofacial trauma, retropharyngeal hematoma	Lymphangioma (cystic hygroma) juvenile nasopharyngeal angiofibroma, tongue neoplasia, neurogenic nasal tumor, teratoma	Myxedema	Central sleep apnea	Burn or inhallational injury, Wegener's, obesity, allergic rhinitis
Supraglottic	Laryngomalacia	Epiglottitis, supraglottitis	Stenosis, intubation injury	Neoplasia			Angioedema, sarcoidosis, burn or inhallational injury
Glottic	Laryngeal stenosis, glottic webbing, laryngeal cleft, laryngeal atresia, vocal cord paralysis/paresis	Laryngitis, diphtheria, tuberculosis	Laryngeal fracture or soft tissue injury, stenosis, foreign body	Neoplasia, respiratory papillomatosis		Vocal cord paralysis/paresis	Hereditary angioedema, burn or inhallational injury
Subglottic	Subglottic stenosis, tracheoesophageal fistulae, vascular sling or ring, aortic arch abnormalities	Laryngotracheal bronchitis	Subglottic stenosis	Neoplasia, fibroma, hemangioma, papilloma	Thyromegaly	Respiratory muscle paralysis	Wegener's
Tracheobronchial	Tracheal stenosis, tracheomalacia, bronchogenic cyst, vascular ring, bronchial web	Tracheitis, bronchitis, tuberculosis	Chronic obstructive pulmonary disease	Neoplasia, fibroma	Goiter		Asthma, burn or inhallational injury

---

Box 2. Modified Malampati

1. Clearly visible tonsils, tonsillar pillars, and soft palate
2. Only visible uvula, tonsillar pillars, upper tonsillar pole
3. Partially visible soft palate
4. Only visible hard palate

Anatomic differences between the adult and pediatric populations include larynx location in the neck, increased airway collapsibility (which attributes to easy obstruction in younger patients), size of occipital bones, relative tongue size, decreased functional pulmonary reserve, and less developed accessory muscles of respiration. The pediatric airway is much smaller than the adult airway in all dimensions including diameter. As the area of the circle is equal to the square of the radius, a very small change in the radius will result in dramatic changes in the patency of the airway. These factors and others help explain why tolerance of apnea and hypoxia is low in infants and children and why situations may quickly sour in a difficult pediatric airway situation. Of note, as a child grows, laryngeal anatomy continually changes; therefore, successful intubation at one point in time does not guarantee future success.

Predictors of a significantly difficult or impossible intubation in pediatric patients include small mouth aperture, hyomental distance 1.5 cm or less in a newborn or infant and 3 cm or less in a child, head and neck impaired mobility (especially in certain syndromes, eg, Downs, juvenile rheumatoid arthritis, Goldenhar), micrognathia, retrognathia, mandibular dysplasia/ hypoplasia, macroglossia, space occupying airway lesions, supra-laryngeal inflammatory pathology, nasal airway obstruction, pathologic obesity, and craniofacial abnormalities [20].

Imaging studies

Radiographic studies may be diagnostic. A chest radiograph may detect a foreign body or large airway obstruction. A CT or MRI of the neck and chest may identify structural causes for airway impairment.

Urgent

Emergent airway cases warrant a concurrent history and physical with careful analysis of acquired information when possible. In an emergent life-threatening situation, the history and physical examination should be undertaken simultaneously. An adult may tolerate slight airway impairment and while a child may initially accommodate to an inadequate airway, increased work required for respiration will recruit accessory muscles until a state of exhaustion is reached or until the airway becomes too narrow to support respiration. The impending respiratory compromise mandates immediate securing of the airway. Since stridor is a symptom and not a diagnosis, a systematic approach must be taken to quickly reach an accurate conclusion (Box 3). Acute stridor may be brought about by an upper respiratory illness exacerbating an underlying anomaly affecting the airway. Additionally, esophageal foreign bodies may push anteriorly against the trachea and impinge upon the airway.

Flexible laryngoscopy may be of immediate assistance during airway evaluation. This should include visualization of bilateral nasal cavities, the nasopharynx, and laryngeal anatomy.

Equipment

Every operating room should be equipped with a dedicated airway management equipment cart. This should be in a location that is readily available and contain instruments for both adult and pediatric patients. Standard equipment should include rigid laryngoscope in multiple sizes with both straight and curved blades, cuffed endotracheal tubes ranging from 2.0 to 8 mm ID, CO_2 detector, tracheal introducer, malleable stylet, Magill forceps in adult and pediatric sizes, laryngeal mask airway (LMA) devices in multiple sizes, face masks for adult and pediatric patients, and a cricothyrotomy set. Additional equipment that may be needed includes flexible fiber-optic scope and light source, nasal trumpet, oral airway, and high-frequency jet ventilator. These devices should be properly maintained and checked for functionality. A dedicated pediatric airway cart should also be readily available.

Across hospitals and emergency rooms, a wide variety of equipment and instrument availability is encountered. This may be because of a lack of clinical data supporting the benefit of one approach over another, operator preference, equipment cost and maintenance required, skill and training of staff, and potential related complications [21].

Management

The goal of difficult airway management is rapid control and correction of an impending airway obstruction. Our philosophy of management should be pessimistic and include Murphy's dictum that "anything that can go

---

Box 3. Stridor mnemonic

S: severity of subjective impression regarding the severity of the obstruction
P: progression of symptoms
E: eating or feeding difficulties, aspiration
C: cyanotic episodes
S: sleep, any obstruction affecting sleep
R: radiology, specific abnormalities detected

wrong will go wrong." We must be prepared for all possibilities. While no universally accepted standard for management of the difficult airway exists, multiple recommendations have been published mostly in the anesthesia literature [5,22–28]. Adaptation of a standardized algorithm of which the anesthesiologist and otolaryngologists agree will lead to the best outcome [29]. It should be kept as simple as possible and use a single dependable piece of equipment for each step of the escalation of treatment. As soon as one method is deemed impracticable, practitioners must quickly advance through the algorithm rather than persist in futile attempts.

In the operative theater, the decision of management may be affected by the type of procedure to be performed and the indication for the procedure. An elective procedure on a patient with a difficult airway may be postponed, performed under local anesthesia or monitored anesthesia care, or the patient may undergo awake fiber-optic intubation. If the desire is to pursue general anesthesia in an elective procedure for a patient with a difficult airway, a skilled anesthesiologist should be available, proper oxygenation should be maintained at all times, and reoxygenation and reevaluation should be performed between repeated intubation attempts. In situations where difficulty exceeds the capabilities of available resources, and if management is deferrable, transfer of the patient to a specialized facility is appropriate. Evaluation of a pediatric patient with a difficult airway is ideally performed during spontaneous respiration without muscle relaxants [20]. Administration of atropine before induction reduces secretions and helps manage bradycardia and preoxygenation with 100% oxygen via face mask for several minutes is routine. In pediatric patients with upper airway obstruction and viral croup, the use of Heliox has proven effective in some cases. Helium is of lower density than the nitrogen found in air, and thus, its use instead of nitrogen decreases airway resistance, lessens the work of respiration, and may help alleviate oxygenation deficits secondary to obstruction.

Securing control of the difficult airway for general anesthesia

In general, we should always anticipate that the present method of obtaining a secure airway will not be successful and always be ready to advance through the algorithm of management options. The following series of modalities used to access the airway is presented in an escalating fashion from standard to more invasive methods.

Mask ventilation

Mask ventilation is an essential element of airway management and is used during induction of general anesthesia before intubation and as a rescue technique during unsuccessful attempts at laryngoscopy and intubation. Hyperoxygenation of a patient by vigorous mask ventilation provides adequate time for intubation or contemplation of the approach to the airway. The mask does not protect from aspiration and when high pressures are required, air may become forced into the esophagus or stomach, elevating the diaphragm and further impairing respiration. Mask ventilation is more difficult in the bearded patient. Insertion of a nasal trumpet or oral airway may augment mask ventilation when there is soft tissue collapse in the upper airway. We should be reluctant to paralyze a patient in whom mask ventilation is difficult.

Tracheal intubation

When the patient is prepared for intubation, standard laryngoscopy is performed and if the airway is visualized, the tracheal tube is inserted. If the airway is not adequately seen, the patient is placed into the modified Jackson's position, external laryngeal pressure is applied and the laryngoscope is maneuvered to improve visualization. Often, these three steps during conventional laryngoscopy provide adequate exposure for direct visualization of the true vocal cords to allow for securing of the airway. If difficulty is encountered during laryngoscopy, one may initially choose to use a larger laryngoscope blade, flexible endotracheal tube stylet, and/ or a magill forceps. If unsuccessful, the practitioner should analyze the cause for not being able to visualize the vocal folds. After three failed attempts at conventional laryngoscopy, it should be abandoned and the physician should proceed with alternative approaches [22,30,31]. Prolonged, persistent repeated laryngoscopy and intubation attempts have been demonstrated to cause laryngeal bleeding, increased secretions, and increasing edema resulting in further inability to adequately ventilate [20]. Ultimately, poor management will lead to hypoxia and significant morbidity or mortality [1,32].

Intubation over flexible bronchoscope

The next choice in a difficult airway may be awake fiber-optic intubation using topical anesthesia. During the attempt, the surgeon is advised to be present in the operating room prepared to perform a tracheotomy if the situation becomes compromised. The flexible bronchoscope is first passed through the endotracheal tube and then through an anesthetized nare or the oral cavity and into the trachea of the awake patient. The mandible and tongue should be pulled strongly anteriorly to expose the larynx. The bronchoscope serves as a visual guide into the trachea and also as a stylet for introduction of the endotracheal tube into the trachea to confirm its placement above the carina. A very thin flexible bronchoscope may become doubled upon itself and even displaced out of the trachea by an endotracheal tube determined to travel into the esophagus. Awake fiber-optic intubation is a safe method to secure a difficult airway, however it requires a cooperative patient [33]. Thus, it is of little use with small children and patients who are uncooperative or combative.

Semi-rigid gum elastic bougie

An anterior commissure laryngoscope, preferably slotted, may be introduced through the corner of the mouth and lateral to the tongue to visualize the larynx (Fig. 1). A semi-rigid gum elastic bougie may then be inserted into the trachea under direct visualization to facilitate introduction of the tube. A tracheal tube then may be inserted over the bougie, which serves as a guide into the trachea.

Laryngeal mask airway

Laryngeal mask airway (LMA) is a well-described instrument for airway control [32,34,35]. This balloon-rimmed mask distributes uniform pressure onto the vallecula, lateral hypopharyngeal walls, piriform sinuses, and retrocricoid areas to seal the gastrointestinal tract from the airway. The device is used rather than a tracheal tube during many procedures. It is also used as a rescue technique in the "can't ventilate, can't intubate" patient. The physician may then proceed to tracheotomy if the situation requires such action.

The use of this device may be limited with the need for high positive-pressure ventilation and possibly when the perceived risk for aspiration is high. It is not very useful in cases of subglottic obstruction. Occasionally, excessive pressure might injure the mucosa and even more rarely injure the recurrent laryngeal nerve.

Surgical interventions

When the above-listed modalities are not successful, surgical management of the airway is preferred [36–38]. Indications for tracheotomy

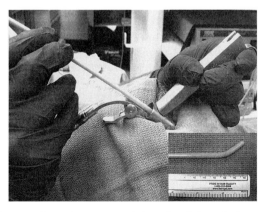

Fig. 1. An anterior commissure laryngoscope is introduced through the corner of the mouth and lateral to the tongue to visualize the larynx. A semi-rigid gum elastic bougie may then be inserted into the trachea under direct visualization to facilitate introduction of the tube (inset image).

were discussed by the American Academy of Otolaryngology Head and Neck surgery in the report entitled "Clinical Indicators Compendium." The list included upper airway obstruction with stridor, bilateral true vocal cord paralysis, previous neck surgery or throat trauma, air hunger, previous radiation to the neck, and accessory muscle use with retractions [39]. Early rapid access to the trachea for adequate ventilation and oxygenation is crucial.

Emergency cricothyrotomy

If the situation deteriorates to "can't ventilate, can't intubate," surgical cricothyrotomy should be quickly performed. Emergency cricothyroidotomy is a time-honored, rapid method for securing the airway and has saved many lives [40,41]. Upon suspicion of the need for a cricothyrotomy tray, it should be brought to the patient's bedside in anticipation of its use. If requirement for the tracheotomy will be prolonged, conversion to a standard tracheotomy within 24 to 48 hours is advisable [37,42].

Elective tracheotomy

Elective tracheotomy is feasible when airway obstruction is anticipated but not imminent, or when a physician is planning a procedure in the head and neck that may cause upper airway swelling or obstruction. The advantage of the tracheotomy over a prolonged period of tracheal intubation is that the patient can be ambulatory and does not require sedation.

Emergent awake tracheotomy

Awake tracheotomy is frequently performed in the patient with impending obstruction as a life-saving procedure. This reliable method to secure the airway is associated with a low complication rate [36,43,44]. Altman and colleagues [36] recommended avoidance of respiratory depressants during the procedure. Ideally the patient will be placed into a semirecumbent position with shoulder roll. A local anesthetic is injected into the overlying skin and strap muscles. A vertical incision is made through skin and midline dissection quickly exposes the trachea and the airway is entered. Once the tracheotomy tube position is confirmed, intravenous anesthetics or paralytics may be delivered [36].

Percutaneous tracheotomy

Several kits are available for this procedure. Familiarity with the specific kit and its use is crucial before actual application in a difficult airway scenario. While some authors suggest this as an option in the emergent setting [45], we believe standard open tracheotomy is preferable as a safe and reliable approach to patients with imminent airway obstruction. Percutaneous tracheotomy requires more time than the poorly oxygenated patient can often supply; however, it may be a useful approach in one's armamentarium for the already ventilated patient in the intensive care unit.

Management by level of obstruction

Oral cavity or hypopharynx

Masses of the oral cavity or pharynx or swelling from nearby abscesses may prevent standard intubation and use of the LMA. In this instance, tracheotomy is the safest method of airway control. Patients with extensive fractures of the facial bones causing prolapse of the tongue and airway impairment may be intubated in the standard approach. If the condition is rapidly reversible, as in the case of an abscess, intubation for a day or two is indicated, but if treatment is prolonged, a tracheotomy allows the patient to be ambulatory and to provide self-care.

Supraglottic level

Swelling or masses may prevent ventilation by mask or LMA and make intubation difficult or impossible. When flexible fiber-optic endoscopy reveals that intubation or LMA is difficult, local tracheotomy provides the safest and most reliable airway.

Glottic level

Preoperative flexible fiber-optic laryngoscopy and CT scans should inform us whether standard intubation or LMA is feasible. If not, tracheotomy is indicated. If the required treatment is prolonged over weeks or longer, tracheotomy is generally warranted.

Subglottic level

CT scans and flexible fiber-optic laryngoscopy should determine whether intubation is feasible. If not, tracheotomy is indicated.

Cervical trachea

Lesions or stenosis below the level of a tracheotomy may be difficult to manage. If the airway is too small for a tracheal tube, a jet ventilator may be the only feasible way to deliver an anesthetic until the tracheal lesion can be resected.

Summary

Otolaryngologists frequently assess and treat difficult airways with the goal of safe and effective management. Knowledge regarding evaluation and management strategies for the difficult airway are crucial. Educational programs to manage the difficult airway should be a part of the training in residency programs, schools of nursing, and for other individuals who may encounter a situation in which knowledge of an airway is required. While a wide variety of equipment is available, we recommend an airway cart be well maintained with sufficient instrumentation for both adult and pediatric airway management. Practitioners should be familiar with the contents of the cart and their application.

Summary of key points

- Difficult airways present in a variety of arenas including the emergency room, operating theater, intensive care unit, procedural suite, and outside of the hospital.
- Knowledge of both adult and pediatric airways regarding anatomy, physical examination findings, and the ability to generate a differential diagnosis assists with preparation for management.
- The availability of adult and pediatric airway equipment is vital for management and intervention and should be well maintained and stored in an early accessible location.
- Management options for the difficult airway include supraglottic maneuvers, tracheal intubations, and surgical interventions.
- The practitioner who anticipates every airway might become challenging will likely always be prepared when the situation becomes compromised.
- Management of a difficult airway may become quite challenging and compromise may quickly evolve necessitating quick intervention.

References

[1] Caplan RA, Benumof JL, Berry FA, et al. Practice guidelines for management of the difficult airway. Anesthesiology 2003;98:1269–77.
[2] Cormack RS, Lehane J. Difficult tracheal intubation in obstetrics. Anaesthesia 1984;39(11): 1105–11.
[3] Cheney FW, Posner KL, Lee LA, et al. Trends in anesthesia-related death and brain damage: a closed claims analysis. Anesthesiology 2006;105(6):1081–6.
[4] Cheney FW. Changing trends in anesthesia-related death and permanent brain damage. ASA Newsl 2002;66(6). Available at: http://depts.washington.edu/asaccp/ASA/Newsletters/asa66_6_6_8.pdf. Accessed January 1, 2007.
[5] Crosby ET, Cooper RM, Douglas MJ, et al. The unanticipated difficult airway with recommendations for management. Can J Anaesth 1998;45:757–76.
[6] Tayal VS, Riggs RW, Marx JA, et al. Rapid-sequence intubation at an emergency medicine residency: success rate and adverse events during a two-year period. Acad Emerg Med 1999;6: 31–7.
[7] Sakles JC, Laurin EG, Rantapaa AA, et al. Airway management in the emergency department: a one-year study of 610 tracheal intubations. Ann Emerg Med 1998;31: 325–32.
[8] Petrini F, Accorsi A, Adrario E, et al. Gruppo di Studio SIAARTI "Vie Aeree Difficili"; IRC e SARNePI; Task Force. Recommendations for airway control and difficult airway management. Minerva Anestesiol 2005;71(11):617–57.
[9] Rocke DA, Murray WB, Rout CC, et al. Relative risk analysis of factors associated with difficult intubation in obstetric anesthesia. Anesthesiology 1992;77:67–73.
[10] El-Gcmzouri AR, McCarthy RJ, Tuman KJ, et al. Preoperative airway assessment: predictive value of a multivariate risk index. Anesth Analg 1996;82:1197–204.
[11] Wilson ME, Spiegelhalter D, Robertson JA, et al. Predicting difficult intubation. Br J Anaesth 1988;61:211–6.
[12] Tse JC, Rimm EB, Hussain A. Predicting difficult intubation in surgical patients scheduled for general anesthesia: a prospective blind study. Anesth Analg 1995;81:254–8.

[13] Lewis M, Keramati S, Benumof JL, et al. What is the best way to determine oropharyngeal classification and mandibular space length to predict difficult laryngoscopy? Anesthesiology 1994;81:69–75.

[14] Hekiert AM, Mandel J, Mirza N. Laryngoscopies in the obese: predicting problems and optimizing visualization. Ann Otol Rhinol Laryngol 2007;116(4):312–6.

[15] Ezri T, Gewurtz G, Sessler DI, et al. Prediction of difficult laryngoscopy in obese patients by ultrasound quantification of anterior neck soft tissue. Anaesthesia 2003;58(11):1111–4.

[16] Ezri T, Medalion B, Weisenberg M, et al. Increased body mass index per se is not a predictor of difficult laryngoscopy. Can J Anaesth 2003;50(2):179–83.

[17] Juvin P, Lavaut E, Dupont H, et al. Difficult tracheal intubation is more common in obese than in lean patients. Anesth Analg 2003;97:595–600.

[18] Brodsky JB, Lemmens HJ, Brock-Utne JG, et al. Morbid obesity and tracheal intubation. Anesth Analg 2002;94:732–6.

[19] Kheterpal S, Han R, Tremper KK, et al. Incidence and predictors of difficult and impossible mask ventilation. Anesthesiology 2006;105(5):885–91.

[20] Gruppo di Studio SIAARTI "Vie Aeree Difficili", Frova G, Guarino A, Petrini F, et al. Recommendations for airway control and difficult airway management in paediatric patients. Minerva Anestesiol 2006;72(9):723–48.

[21] Levitan RM, Kush S, Hollander JE. Devices for difficult airway management in academic emergency departments: results of a national survey. Ann Emerg Med 1999; 33(6):694–8.

[22] American Society of Anesthesiologists Task Force on Management of the Difficult Airway. Practice guidelines for management of the difficult airway. An updated report. Anesthesiology 2003;95:1269–77.

[23] Braun U, Goldmann K, Hempel V, et al. [Airway management]. Leitlinie der deutschen gesellschaft für anästhesiologie und intensivmedizin. Anaesthesiol Intensivmed Notfallmed Schmerzther 2004;45:302–6 [in German].

[24] Boisson-Bertrand D, Bourgain JL, Camboulives J, et al. Intubation difficile Société française d'anesthésie et de réanimation. Expertise collective. Ann Fr Anesth Réanim 1996;15:207–14 [in French].

[25] SIAARTI Task Force on Difficult Airway Management. L'intubazione difficile e la difficoltà di controllo delle vie aeree nell'adulto (SIAARTI). Minerva Anestesiol 1998;64:361–71, [in English and Italian].

[26] Henderson JJ, Popat M, Latto IP, et al. Difficult Airway Society guidelines for management of the unanticipated difficult intubation. Anaesthesia 2004;59:675–94.

[27] Kelly JT, Toepp MC. Practice parameters: development, evaluation, dissemination, and implementation. QRB Qual Rev Bull 1992;18:405–9.

[28] Walker RD, Howard MO, Lambert MD, et al. Medical practice guidelines. West J Med 1994;161:39–44.

[29] Heidegger T, Gerig HJ, Henderson JJ. Strategies and algorithms for management of the difficult airway. Best Pract Res Clin Anaesthesiol 2005;19(4):661–74.

[30] Mort TC. Emergency tracheal intubation: complications associated with repeated laryngoscopic attempts. Anesth Analg 2004;99:607–13.

[31] Peterson GN, Domino KB, Caplan RA, et al. Management of the difficult airway: a closed claims analysis. Anesthesiology 2005;103:33–9.

[32] Benumof JL. Laryngeal mask airway and the ASA difficult airway algorithm. Anesthesiology 1996;84(3):686–99.

[33] Benumof JL. Management of the difficult adult airway. With special emphasis on awake tracheal intubation. Anesthesiology 1991;75(6):1087–110.

[34] Parmet JL, Colonna-Romano P, Horrow JC, et al. The laryngeal mask airway reliably provides rescue ventilation in cases of unanticipated difficult tracheal intubation along with difficult mask ventilation. Anesth Analg 1998;87(3):661–5.

[35] Combes X, Le Roux B, Suen P, et al. Unanticipated difficult airway in anesthetized pa-
     tients: prospective validation of a management algorithm. Anesthesiology 2004;100(5):
     1146–50.
[36] Altman KW, Waltonen JD, Kern RC. Urgent surgical airway intervention: a 3 year county
     hospital experience. Laryngoscope 2005;115:2101–4.
[37] Yuen HW, Loy AH, Johari S. Urgent awake tracheotomy for impending airway obstruction.
     Otolaryngol Head Neck Surg 2007;136(5):838–42.
[38] McWhorter AJ. Tracheotomy: timing and techniques. Curr Opin Otolaryngol Head Neck
     Surg 2003;11(6):473–9.
[39] Archer SM, Baugh RF, Nelms CR, et al. Tracheostomy. In: 2000 Clinical indicators
     compendium. Alexandria (VA): American Academy of Otolaryngology Head and Neck Sur-
     gery; 2000. p. 45.
[40] Bair AE, Panacek EA, Wisner DH, et al. Cricothyrotomy: a 5-year experience at one
     institution. J Emerg Med 2003;24(2):151–6.
[41] DeLaurier GA, Hawkins ML, Treat RC, et al. Acute airway management. Role of cricothyr-
     oidotomy. Am Surg 1990;56(1):12–5.
[42] Esses BA, Jafek BW. Cricothyroidotomy: a decade of experience in Denver. Ann Otol
     Rhinol Laryngol 1987;96(5):519–24.
[43] Waldron J, Padgham ND, Hurley SE. Complications of emergency and elective tracheos-
     tomy: a retrospective study of 150 consecutive cases. Ann R Coll Surg Engl 1990;72(4):
     218–20.
[44] Gillespie MB, Eisele DW. Outcomes of emergency surgical airway procedures in a hospital-
     wide setting. Laryngoscope 1999;109(11):1766–9.
[45] Ault MJ, Ault B, Ng PK. Percutaneous dilatational tracheostomy for emergent airway
     access. J Intensive Care Med 2003;18(4):222–6.

ELSEVIER
SAUNDERS

Otolaryngol Clin N Am
41 (2008) 581–596

OTOLARYNGOLOGIC
CLINICS
OF NORTH AMERICA

Intraoperative Emergencies During Endoscopic Sinus Surgery: CSF Leak and Orbital Hematoma

Kevin C. Welch, MD, James N. Palmer, MD*

Department of Otorhinolaryngology, Division of Rhinology, University of Pennsylvania Health System, 5 Ravdin, 3400 Spruce Street, Philadelphia, PA 19104, USA

Over the past 20 years, endoscopic sinus surgery has been widely used as a safe and effective treatment for disorders of the paranasal sinuses that are refractory to medical therapy. Advances in surgical technique, including powered instrumentation and stereotactic image-guided surgery, have improved the efficiency and safety of this procedure. Despite these advances, complications are still encountered.

Among the most common risks encountered in endoscopic sinus surgery (eg, bleeding, infection, injury to the eye, cerebrospinal fluid [CSF] leak, anosmia, myocardial infarction, cerebrovascular accident, need for revision surgery), approximately 83% to 100% of patients considered cerebrospinal fluid leak or injury to the eye to be the most important risks warranting discussion. Similarly, catastrophic orbital bleeding and iatrogenic CSF leak are the two serious complications surgeons most fear. However, thorough preoperative planning and meticulous surgical technique can help minimize these risks. Moreover, surgeons managing these complications using a stepwise approach can avoid untoward long-term sequellae.

This article discusses these two avoidable complications and provides treatment algorithms for intraoperative maneuvers.

Intraoperative cerebrospinal fluid leaks

Prevention of intraoperative CSF leaks begins with a thorough understanding of the anatomy of the paranasal sinuses, particularly their relationships with the anterior skull base.

---

* Corresponding author.
E-mail address: james.palmer@uphs.upenn.edu (J.N. Palmer).

0030-6665/08/$ - see front matter © 2008 Elsevier Inc. All rights reserved.
doi:10.1016/j.otc.2008.01.005

Anatomy of the anterior skull base

Surgeons must understand the relationship between the ethmoid sinuses and the anterior skull base. Understanding this relationship begins in the preoperative setting through reviewing CT images of the patient's anatomy. CT imaging must be performed in the coronal plane in all patients before undergoing endoscopic sinus surgery. If available, thin slice (1.0–3.0 mm) axial images reconstructed in the coronal and sagittal planes provided further elucidation of the skull base anatomy.

Coronal images provide crucial information on several critical areas that, if overlooked, can lead to intraoperative complications. On coronal images, the height of the maxillary sinus should be compared with the height of the ethmoid sinuses. The ratio of maxillary-to-ethmoid height (Fig. 1) can vary from 1:1 to 2:1 and can be used preoperatively to guide how dissection through the basal lamella will lead to the anterior skull base along the posterior ethmoid sinuses. Meyers [1] has shown how this ratio can lead to inadvertent injury to the anterior skull base during dissection. The ratio can be further examined along the slope of the skull base, which is best viewed in sagittal or parasagittal images. A line extended from the limen nasi to the basal lamella will identify the distance to which the skull base will be encountered. Additionally, the slope of the skull base from frontal recess to planum sphenoidale will correlate these findings. The thickness of the anterior skull base should also be examined thoroughly with both coronal and sagittal CT images. The thickness of the anterior skull base varies and is often asymmetric in individual patients. Knowing the thickness of the anterior skull base is important, because the roof of the ethmoid has been shown to be the place of least resistance during dissection (Fig. 2) [2]. In addition to its

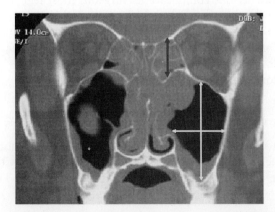

Fig. 1. A coronal CT of a preoperative patient demonstrating a maxillary sinus-to-ethmoid sinus ratio of 2:1. The short ethmoid height serves as an indicator to the surgeon that the anterior skull base will be quickly encountered when the basal lamella is removed before dissection of the posterior ethmoid sinuses.

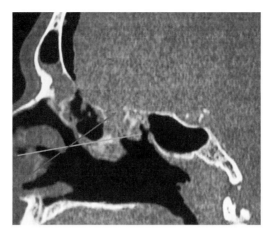

Fig. 2. A sagittal CT of the maxillofacial region in a patient after endoscopic sinus surgery in which the anterior skull base was injured during posterior ethmoid dissection, the point where the skull base is the weakest. This patient had a maxillary sinus-to-ethmoid sinus ratio greater than 1:1. The figure illustrates the "angle of attack" that is directed through the basal lamella.

anatomy, the skull base itself should be examined for areas of dehiscence, thinness, and thickness, and for soft tissue that might suggest an encephalocele.

The region of the ethmoid roof and cribriform plate is of critical importance and is best analyzed in the coronal plane. In the midline of the ethmoid bone is the cribriform plate (*lamina cribrosa*), which represents the lowest point of the skull base in the median aspect of the nasal cavity. Multiple perforations of the cribriform plate permit transmission of neural fibers into the nasal cavity that contribute to olfaction. The lateral mass (or labyrinth) of the ethmoid is suspended laterally from the cribriform plate by the fovea ethmoidalis, or ethmoid roof. Interposed between the cribriform plate and the fovea ethmoidalis is the lateral cribriform lamella. The sagittal buttress of the middle turbinate is suspended from the articulation of the cribriform plate and the lateral cribriform lamella. When viewed in the coronal plane, the three bony structures are said to possess a "gull wing in flight" appearance (Fig. 3); however, this structure has significant variations. Keros and colleagues [3] studied the relationship of these bony structures and proposed a classification based on the length of the lateral cribriform lamella. The classification is as follows: Keros type I (1–3 mm deep), Keros type II (4–7 mm deep), and Keros type III (8–16 mm deep). Ali and colleagues [4] showed that type II anatomy is the most commonly encountered and the symmetry of the olfactory fossa varies widely among patients [4–6]. The classification is useful because patients who have a lower Keros classification are believed to have a lower risk for intracranial injury and those who have a higher Keros classification a higher risk for intracranial injury and postoperative CSF leak.

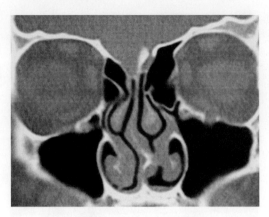

Fig. 3. A coronal CT image of a patient showing a low and asymmetric olfactory fossa. Dissection along the right anterior skull base can lead to inadvertent injury if the surgeon does not recognize the differences in ethmoid height in this patient.

Intraoperative management of cerebrospinal fluid leaks

Despite review of the preoperative films, use of intraoperative stereotactic image-guided surgery, and meticulous surgical technique, a violation of the anterior skull base can occur. If this untoward event occurs, the authors recommend the algorithm provided in Fig. 4 to manage this complication.

When a leak occurs, the surgeon should stop and review the anatomy. Landmarks (eg, posterior wall of the maxillary sinus, attachments of the middle turbinate, anterior face of the sphenoid sinus, skull base) within the patient should be identified to help reorient the surgeon, and then the preoperative and stereotactic imaging should be used to help localize the probable site of the leak. The most likely sites of injury include the lateral cribriform lamella and cribriform plate; therefore, surgeons should review these areas for dehiscences, asymmetries, thinness/thickness, or any bony abnormalities on the preoperative imaging. Additional attention should be directed to the posterior ethmoid sinuses to determine if reduced posterior ethmoid height (ie, maxillary–ethmoid ratio greater than 1:1) is present that would precipitate inadvertent injury to the skull base. If a particular region is suspected, an attempt should be made to correlate the radiographic site with the region endoscopically.

If the site cannot be completely identified or if the operating surgeon does not feel equipped to repair the defect, then adequate hemostasis should be obtained and the nasal cavity lightly packed to help apply gentle pressure to the defect. The surgeon should be aware that the process of gaining hemostasis can actually cause more complications, and the endoscopic view greatly magnifies any blood loss. They should therefore proceed with caution, especially when using monopolar cautery near the skull base. The upper and lower aerodigestive tract should be aspirated for blood and antiemetics administered to minimize postoperative nausea. All efforts should

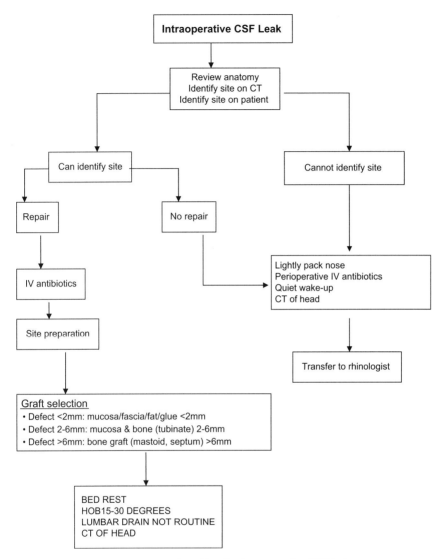

Fig. 4. Algorithm for addressing intraoperative CSF leaks.

be made to minimize increases in intracranial pressure, and particular attention should be directed toward minimizing Valsalva maneuvers during arousal from general anesthesia. If safe, a deep extubation can be performed. Avoidance of nasal positive airway pressure is imperative, despite the extubation plan, because of the potential for pneumocephalus. Immediate head CT is warranted to document that no hematoma or pneumocephalus has occurred, which can be life-threatening.

The efficacy of antibiotic prophylaxis for preventing meningitis in patients who have postsurgical CSF leaks has not been studied in a prospective manner; however, several retrospective reviews of traumatic CSF leaks have yielded conflicting information. A meta-analysis by Brodie and colleagues [7] showed no significant differences in the rates of ascending meningitis in patients treated with and without antibiotics in traumatic anterior skull base CSF leaks. Conversely, Bernal-Sprekelsen and colleagues [8] found an incidence of ascending meningitis in 29% of patients treated conservatively (eg, head of bed elevation, bed rest). Although not statistically significant, 40% of patients treated transcranially also developed meningitis. However, in a separate study, these investigators found an incidence of ascending meningitis in 36.5% of patients undergoing endoscopic repair of CSF leaks. During endoscopic sinus surgery, presumably the anterior skull base is penetrated with an instrument (eg, curette, microdebrider), and bacteria or inflamed or infected mucosa is implanted intracranially, which may contribute to infection. Therefore, the authors believe it is prudent to administer perioperative parenteral antibiotics (eg, ceftriaxone) that effectively cross the blood–brain barrier, because an intraoperative CSF leak by definition includes an element of direct trauma to the brain, however minor.

A subarachnoid lumbar drain has been advocated for planned treatment of CSF leaks. However, no prospective studies have examined the use and duration of lumbar drains in patients who have experienced iatrogenic endoscopic sinus surgery injuries. In most instances, the authors believe a lumbar drain is unnecessary for an iatrogenic injury unless the patient has signs of benign intracranial hypertension, empty sella syndrome, or radiographic evidence of dehiscent bone along the skull base that would otherwise suggest elevated intracranial pressures.

Finally, transfer of service to a local rhinologist is recommended for continued care of the patient. Operating surgeons should proceed with closure only after they have identified the site of leak, understand the anatomy, and are prepared to attempt closure, and the patients are stable.

Transnasal endoscopic repair of CSF leaks has been reported to be successful in 90% to 97% of patients [9,10] during a first attempt. Once the site of the leak is identified and prepared, surgeons should adhere to three goals: (1) safe and successful closure of the leak; (2) maintenance of sinus function; and (3) prevention of postoperative complications. The major sites of anterior skull base injury are reviewed.

Ethmoid/cribriform leaks

The surgical site is prepared by completing a maxillary antrostomy and total ethmoidectomy with wide exposure of the skull base. If exposure of the defect requires the removal of the middle turbinate, then its resection should be complete to prevent postoperative lateralization of the middle turbinate remnant and iatrogenic frontal recess obstruction. If the middle turbinate is removed, it should be preserved for later use as grafting material. If the repair is likely to cause postoperative obstruction of the frontal recess or the sphenoethmoidal recess, a prophylactic frontal sinusotomy or sphenoidotomy should be performed.

Once the defect is fully delineated, the mucosa surrounding the defect is stripped and potentially fulgurated with bipolar electrocautery 3 to 4 mm beyond the bony defect rim. The authors then size the defect measured using a trimmed ruler. Defects smaller than 2 mm will likely heal with a combination of osteoneogenesis and soft tissue fibrosis; therefore, the authors do not recommend preparing the epidural space or placing a bone graft to avoid increasing the size of the defect. Simple abrasion of the surrounding bone (scraping versus drilling with diamond bur) with placement of an overlay graft (eg, mucosa, temporalis fascia) dressed with a thin layer of fibrin glue sufficiently patches most leaks. Excessive fibrin glue should be avoided to help facilitate remucosalization.

A composite graft is often suited for the repair of defects larger than 2 mm but smaller than 6 mm. In these circumstances, a middle turbinate composite (mucosa/bone) graft is an excellent choice for repair, because the bone of the middle turbinate has similar density to the bone of the cribriform plate and anterior skull base. Resection of the middle turbinate should occur at the skull base to prevent postoperative lateralization of the middle turbinate remnant and iatrogenic stenosis of the frontal recess. Once the turbinate is harvested, it can be filleted and the mucosa stripped from one side. Once the defect is measured, the excess bone of the middle turbinate is removed, taking care to leave behind mucoperiosteum. The appropriately sized middle turbinate bone is then wedged into the defect, allowing the periosteum to be applied to the cleaned skull base and the mucosa facing the nasal cavity.

Defects larger than 6 mm are closed in a multilayered fashion with underlay bone grafting to reconstitute the native skull base anatomy (Fig. 5).

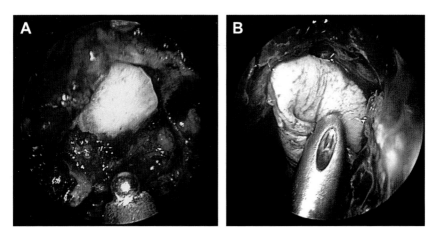

Fig. 5. Endoscopic view of an anterior skull base defect that is repaired with mastoid cortex bone as an underlay graft (*A*) and with septal mucosa as an overlay (*B*) graft.

Septal bone and mastoid cortex are two choices for bone grafting. The advantages of septal bone include its ease of access intranasally and the osteoneogenic properties of the overlying mucoperichondrium. Care must be taken when harvesting the septal bone, because iatrogenic septal perforations may result; furthermore, portions of the septal bone may be fairly flimsy and fracture easily during placement. In situations of poor septal bone, the authors recommend using mastoid cortex, because sufficient bone is available for contouring, and soft tissue (eg, fascia, muscle) can be obtained for additional layered support. Harvesting mastoid cortex, however, requires a separate incision and site preparation, which may increase intraoperative time. The final defect size should be measured and the mucosa surrounding the defect stripped and potentially fulgurated. The dura is elevated using a round knife, ball-tipped seeker, or other appropriate instrument, and the bone graft is placed in an underlay fashion. Fibrin glue is applied lightly, and a pliable soft tissue graft (eg, fascia, mucosa) is placed as an overlay and secured with a thin coating of fibrin glue.

Sphenoid sinus cerebrospinal leaks

Leaks within the sphenoid sinus may occur during transsphenoidal hypophysectomy or during routine endoscopic sinus surgery. In these instances, fat grafting used as an onlay graft or as biologic packing to reinforce a fascial graft works well to seal midline sphenoid sinus leaks. Additionally, middle turbinate composite grafts work well to close the moderate-sized, midline sphenoid sinus CSF leak. Care must be taken during preparation to not strip the sphenoid sinus mucosa too far laterally, because this will place the optic nerve and carotid artery at a great risk for injury.

Frontal sinus cerebrospinal leaks

CSF leaks involving the frontal sinus require the most skill to repair. These leaks can be separated into those involving the frontal sinus posterior table, frontal recess, or anterior ethmoid adjacent to the outflow tract. The type of repair will depend on the location, extent of preparation, and graft selection. A wide frontal sinusotomy should be performed (if it was not previously) to prevent outflow obstruction of the frontal sinus after a repair. Any supraorbital ethmoid, agger nasi, and frontal recess cells should be widely opened so that postoperative stenosis of the frontal sinus outflow tract is avoided. If the injury or site preparation extends too far superiorly or laterally, the repair may require the assistance of a trephination or an osteoplastic flap for definitive repair. Therefore, this repair may be best left for another time or after transfer to a rhinologist.

Once prepared, the site is repaired using similar principles as described earlier. The main differences involve the use of the 70° endoscope and instrumentation (eg, frontal sinus curette, giraffe forceps) designed for the frontal sinus. A frontal sinus stent composed of thin Silastic sheeting is placed to stabilize the graft and help maintain frontal sinus patency postoperatively. This stent is removed 1 week postoperatively. Woodworth and colleagues [11] treated seven patients who had CSF leaks originating from the frontal sinus and frontal recess using these principles, all of whom were treated successfully during the first attempt and maintained long-term frontal recess patency.

Summary

Preoperative planning and meticulous surgical technique involving the use of state-of-the-art instrumentation can help improve the efficiency and safety of endoscopic sinus surgery. When an intraoperative leak is encountered, surgeons must assess the damage and decide to stop or proceed based on their experience and resources. Proper site preparation, graft selection, and preservation of outflow tracts are essential for success. As with the conservative management algorithm, patients who undergo an intraoperative repair of an iatrogenic CSF leak should receive perioperative intravenous antibiotics (eg, ceftriaxone) and be placed on short-term bed rest. A lumbar drain is not necessary for an iatrogenic leak unless signs of increased intracranial pressure are present. A lumbar drain in this instance with the possible adjuvant administration of acetazolamide, 500 mg twice daily, can help relieve pressure on the repair, because increased CSF pressure often affects postoperative management.

Intraoperative bleeding: orbital hematoma

Blood loss during endoscopic sinus surgery can vary depending on the pathology, surgical technique, and choice of anesthesia. Although the pathology may not be controlled, preoperative planning and technique can greatly improve outcomes and minimize bleeding complications.

Anatomy of the orbit and anterior ethmoid artery

The orbit itself is comprised of seven bones: maxilla, zygoma, frontal, lacrimal, sphenoid, palatine, and ethmoid. These bones form a conical-shaped cavity that is approximately 3.5 to 4.0 cm wide and 4.5 to 5.0 cm long. The extraocular muscles are suspended from the orbital bones and various suspensory ligaments, which support the globe. The thickness of the orbital walls varies but is generally thinnest along the orbital floor and the medial aspect of the orbit, generally less than 1 mm.

The medial aspect of the orbit is known as the *lamina papyracea*, and the bone itself is the lateral-most extension of the ethmoid bone. This thin bony layer is another critical anatomic structure that must be examined preoperatively and identified intraoperatively. The thickness, contour, and presence of infraorbital (Haller) or supraorbital cells should be identified. Although bony dehiscences in the lamina papyracea are uncommon [12], the full length of the lamina papyracea should be examined for their occurrences. Defects in the lamina papyracea resulting from previous maxillofacial trauma should also be identified because they may appear similar to ethmoidal air cells in the endoscopic setting or may hinder the dissection of posterior ethmoid sinuses.

At the apex of the orbit is the optic canal, which permits passage of the optic nerve and ophthalmic artery, from which arise the anterior and posterior ethmoid arteries. These vessels perforate the nasal cavity through the frontoethmoidal suture and travel in grooves along the surface of the horizontal portion of the ethmoid bone.

The anterior ethmoid artery is a critical structure to identify when clearing the skull base and opening the frontal recess. Moon and colleagues [13] performed an extensive dissection of cadaveric heads and found that the anterior ethmoidal canal was 49 ± 4.9 mm from the limen nasi at an angle of 54.5° ± 6.8°. They also determined that the anterior ethmoidal canal was located between the second and third lamella in 87% of cadavers, within the third lamella in 11%, and within the second lamella in 2%. In 91% of cadavers, the anterior ethmoidal canal was located either within the skull base or protruded 2 to 3 mm below the skull base; in 8.5%, the anterior ethmoidal canal was suspended in a bony mesentery. Close inspection of sagittal CT images will show the anterior ethmoidal canal within a bony swelling of the skull base between the second and third lamella. Coronal CT images perhaps allow visualization of a more useful landmark for locating the anterior ethmoidal artery; a bony "nipple" occurring at the confluence of the medial rectus and superior oblique muscles indicates the nasal origin of the anterior ethmoidal artery (Fig. 6). This bony structure can be seen on preoperative CT images to help identify a potential source of significant bleeding during complete dissection along the skull base. Moreover, through using stereotactic image-guided surgery, this landmark can be continually reassessed intraoperatively during dissection to help avoid bleeding complications.

The pattern of posterior ethmoid and sphenoid pneumatization should be examined before any endoscopic sinus surgery. It is essential to establish whether a sphenoethmoidal (ie, Onodi) cell is present. The precise definition of an Onodi cell has changed since its original description in 1910 [14] of the variation of posterior ethmoid pneumatization; however, this cell, which occurs in 8% to 14% of the general population, is now considered to be a posterior ethmoid cell that pneumatizes lateral and superior to the sphenoid sinus [15]. Although Onodi cells are typically associated with the optic nerve, it is not required. These two aspects of the Onodi cell make its identification crucial before dissecting out the posterior ethmoids. Mistaking the Onodi cell for the sphenoid sinus can lead to incomplete dissection and place the optic nerve at risk and further injure the orbit.

The optic nerve typically forms an indentation in the lateral wall of the sphenoid sinus, and approximately 5% of these have dehiscent bone; this can occur unilaterally or bilaterally. Additionally, the carotid artery can

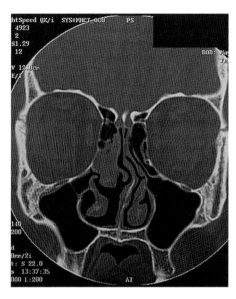

Fig. 6. The anterior ethmoid artery canal can be located at the confluence of the superior oblique muscle and the medial rectus muscle as a "nipple" on coronal CT imaging.

also indent the lateral sphenoid sinus wall, with 7% of these being dehiscent. Inspection of the posterosuperior portion of the sphenoid sinus will typically reveal the opticocarotid recess or the confluence of these two structures. Preoperative imaging reviewed in the axial plane will show excellent detail of the sphenoid sinus and its relationships with the optic nerve (traced back from the orbit) and carotid artery. Often septations within the sphenoid sinus will insert on the bony canal of the carotid artery. Identifying these structures preoperatively and intraoperatively helps reduce injuries.

Intraoperative management of orbital bleeding

Prevention of intraoperative bleeding begins with an appropriate preoperative history and physical examination, with appropriate attention to the patient's medical history; bleeding history; use of antiplatelet or anticoagulant therapy; use of over-the-counter herbal or alternative medicines, such as ginkgo, garlic, and ginseng; and hematocrit, hemoglobin, platelet count, and coagulation factors (eg, prothrombin time, international normalized ratio, partial thromboplastin time) status. If medically safe, antiplatelet therapies should be ceased at least 10 days before endoscopic sinus surgery.

Preparation of the nasal cavity before surgery is essential. The mucosa should be decongested with pledgets moistened with oxymetazoline, phenylephrine, or cocaine solution for at least 10 minutes before performing endoscopy. Injections with 1% lidocaine with 1:100,000 (1:200,000 if increased cardiac risk) epinephrine should then be placed transorally into the greater palatine foramina to address the sphenopalatine artery and intranasally at the root of the middle turbinate and at the inferior body of the middle turbinate. If the sphenopalatine injection is not performed transorally, it may be performed transnasally at the site of the sphenopalatine foramen near the lateral attachment of the middle turbinate. In conjunction with total intravenous anesthesia [16], relative hypotension, and relative bradycardia, these efforts can help minimize intraoperative blood loss while simultaneously improving visualization and preventing intraoperative complications.

A compliment of instruments, topical decongestants, and prothrombotic agents should be readily available to the surgeon so that potential intraoperative bleeding may be addressed. The authors recommend monopolar suction cautery, bipolar cautery, pledgets moistened with 10,000 units of thrombin mixed with 1:10,000 epinephrine, Avitene microfibrillar collagen slurry, and sponge packing.

Orbital hematomas can occur rapidly or slowly, depending on whether the injury is venous or arterial [17]. Despite the cause, orbital hematomas constitute an ophthalmologic emergency, because an intraorbital bleed can rapidly produce an orbital compartment syndrome with permanent injury to the optic nerve if ischemia time is greater than 90 minutes.

Injury to the lamina papyracea with bleeding from periorbita, ocular fat, or extraocular muscles can occur with aggressive dissection along the lamina papyracea with powered instrumentation or inattention to anatomic variations. When the lamina papyracea is violated, inspection for periorbita and periorbital fat should be undertaken. If the periorbita is not violated and no signs of orbital injury are present, the surgeon can decide to stop or proceed if the prolapsing orbital contents have not caused significant obstruction. If the periorbita is cut and orbital fat is exposed, an intraoperative ophthalmology consult should be obtained to measure intraocular pressures and perform forced duction testing if required. Early signs of an orbital hematoma include preseptal edema, ecchymosis, orbital proptosis, and raised intraocular pressures (normal range, 10–20 mm Hg). The speed at which these signs occur may help indicate whether a slow venous bleed or an arterial bleed is the cause. If intraocular pressures are normal, the eye should be continually observed and reassessed until the patient emerges from anesthesia and a visual acuity examination can be performed (Fig. 7). If intraocular pressures are elevated, massage of the eye, administration of mannitol at 1 to 2 g/kg over 30 minutes as a 15% to 25% solution, and administration of 10 mg of intravenous dexamethasone is indicated. In the awake patient, timolol, 0.5%, at 1 to 2 drops twice daily can help reduce intraocular pressures through decreasing the production of aqueous humor. These conservative measures may fail to reduce intraocular pressures acutely; therefore, the surgeon and ophthalmologist must decide whether to observe the patient or pursue more aggressive treatment. Absolute indications for canthotomy/ cantholysis in the anesthetized patient include intraocular pressures greater than 40 mm Hg. In the awake patient, additional confirming signs that

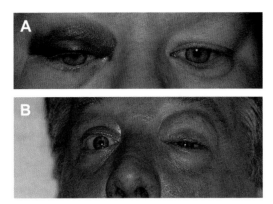

Fig. 7. (*A*) A patient who sustained an anterior ethmoid artery injury during endoscopic sinus surgery. Fortunately, orbital complications were limited to the preseptal subcutaneous tissues. Ocular testing was otherwise normal. (*B*) The result of intraconal air in a patient who has an injury to the lamina papyracea.

direct one to performing a canthotomy/cantholysis include severe retroorbital pain, Marcus-Gunn pupil, and a cherry red macula.

A lateral canthotomy (Fig. 8) is performed after 1% lidocaine with 1:100,000 epinephrine is administered to the lateral canthus. A hemostat

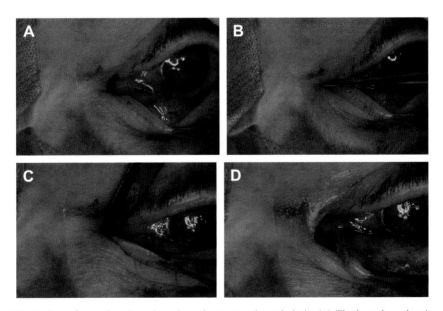

Fig. 8. Steps for performing a lateral canthotomy and cantholysis. (*A*) The lateral canthus is incised beginning with the lateral lid commissure. (*B*) Retraction of the inferior lid shows the extent of the incision. (*C*) The inferior crus of the lateral canthal tendon is divided. (*D*) The lower lid and canthal tendon are retracted to show the final result. (*Courtesy of* R. Gausas, MD, Philadelphia, PA).

may be used to crimp the skin of the lateral canthus to further assist with hemostasis. Next, a 1- to 2-cm incision from the lateral commissure through the lateral canthus is performed, which will typically instantaneously reduce intraocular pressures on the globe by approximately 14 mm Hg [18]. However, the release of pressure may not be sufficient, and a cantholysis should be performed. The superior and inferior portions of the lateral canthal tendon attach to Whitnall's tubercle, which lies 4 mm posterior to the lateral orbital rim of the zygomatic bone. Fine scissors are used to release the inferior portion of the lateral canthal tendon to complete the cantholysis. Releasing the lateral canthal tendon reduces intraocular pressures an additional 19 mm Hg [18]. The canthotomy may be repaired later when the intraocular pressures are clearly normal.

Once the globe is addressed, the source of bleeding should be identified. If no bleeding is observed, blind cautery of the periorbital fat should be avoided to prevent injury to the extraocular muscles and optic nerve. However, if bleeding is observed and does not involve the orbit itself, bipolar electrocautery works well. When an arterial bleed occurs in isolation of an orbital injury, the most likely culprit is the anterior ethmoidal artery, which can be easily encountered posterior to the frontal recess between the second and third lamella and identified on preoperative imaging. Typically, this artery is located within the skull base; however, it can project from the skull base or be located in a bony mesentery that may be mistaken as a simple ethmoid lamella. When an injury occurs, the artery can retract into the orbit, causing rapid hemorrhage into a confined space, and the patient can manifest signs of orbital hematoma. This complication is less likely to occur with the posterior ethmoid artery because of its location near the anterior roof of the sphenoid and its less-accessible canal. In this instance, rapid control of the bleeding with attention to the previously recommended steps (massage, mannitol, ophthalmology consultation, canthotomy/cantholysis) is indicated. If necessary, external incisions may be necessary to ligate the anterior and posterior ethmoid arteries if they cannot be addressed endoscopically. Postoperatively, a CT of the orbits is indicated to assess the status of the globe.

Summary

Intraoperative orbital hematoma constitutes an emergency, and improper management can lead to permanent blindness. Thorough preoperative planning and careful dissection help reduce the risk for orbital injury; however, if an injury occurs, a stepwise approach (Fig. 9), the timely administration of intravenous medications, and the appropriate use of canthotomy with or without cantholysis can reduce complications related to an orbital compartment syndrome. Short- and long-term consultation with an ophthalmologist is indicated for serial visual acuity examinations and continuity of care.

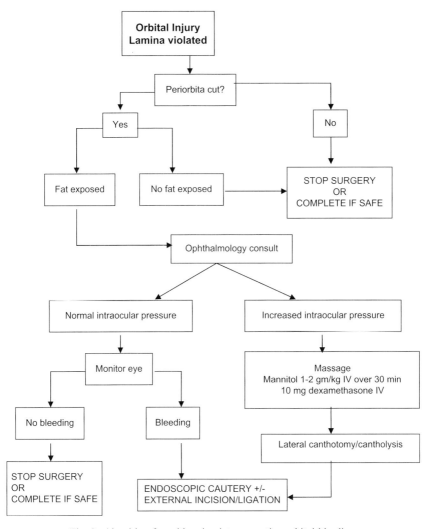

Fig. 9. Algorithm for addressing intraoperative orbital bleeding.

Summary

Patient safety and health is the most important factor during endoscopic sinus surgery. It is better to stop a surgery and proceed at a later date or refer the patient to a rhinologist than to continue under suboptimal conditions. The two most feared complications related to endoscopic sinus surgery, CSF leaks and orbital hematomas, are preventable. However, when they occur, a stepwise approach to therapy can assure consistent treatment.

References

[1] Meyers RM, Valvassori G. Interpretation of anatomic variations of computed tomography scans of the sinuses: a surgeon's perspective. Laryngoscope 1998;108:422–5.

[2] Kainz J, Stammberger H. The roof of the anterior ethmoid: a locus minoris resistentiae in the skull base). Laryngol Rhinol Otol (Stuttg) 1988;67:142–9 [in German].

[3] Keros P. On the practical value of differences in the level of the lamina cribrosa of the ethmoid). Z Laryngol Rhinol Otol 1962;41:809–13 [in German].

[4] Ali A, Kurien M, Shyamkumar NK. Anteiror skull base: high risk areas in endoscopic sinus surgery in chronic rhinosinusitis: a computed tomographic anaylsis. Indian J Otolaryngol Head Neck Surg 2005;57:5–8.

[5] Lebowitz RA, Terk A, Jacobs JB, et al. Asymmetry of the ethmoid roof: analysis using coronal computed tomography. Laryngoscope 2001;111:2122–4.

[6] Dessi P, Moulin G, Triglia JM, et al. Difference in the height of the right and left ethmoidal roofs: a possible risk factor for ethmoidal surgery. Prospective study of 150 CT scans. J Laryngol Otol 1994;108:261–2.

[7] Brodie HA. Prophylactic antibiotics for posttraumatic cerebrospinal fluid fistulae. A meta-analysis. Arch Otolaryngol Head Neck Surg 1997;123:749–52.

[8] Bernal-Sprekelsen M, Bleda-Vazquez C, Carrau RL. Ascending meningitis secondary to traumatic cerebrospinal fluid leaks. Am J Rhinol 2000;14:257–9.

[9] Lanza DC, O'Brien DA, Kennedy DW. Endoscopic repair of cerebrospinal fluid fistulae and encephaloceles. Laryngoscope 1996;106:1119–25.

[10] Hegazy HM, Carrau RL, Snyderman CH, et al. Transnasal endoscopic repair of cerebrospinal fluid rhinorrhea: a meta-analysis. Laryngoscope 2000;110:1166–72.

[11] Woodworth BA, Schlosser RJ, Palmer JN. Endoscopic repair of frontal sinus cerebrospinal fluid leaks. J Laryngol Otol 2005;119:709–13.

[12] Moulin G, Dessi P, Chagnaud C, et al. Dehiscence of the lamina papyracea of the ethmoid bone: CT findings. AJNR Am J Neuroradiol 1994;15:151–3.

[13] Moon HJ, Kim HU, Lee JG, et al. Surgical anatomy of the anterior ethmoidal canal in ethmoid roof. Laryngoscope 2001;111:900–4.

[14] Onodi A. The optic nerve and the accessory sinuses of the nose. New York: William Wood & Co.; 1910.

[15] Stammberger HR, Kennedy DW. Paranasal sinuses: anatomic terminology and nomenclature. The Anatomic Terminology Group. Ann Otol Rhinol Laryngol Suppl 1995;167:7–16.

[16] Wormald PJ, van Renen G, Perks J, et al. The effect of the total intravenous anesthesia compared with inhalational anesthesia on the surgical field during endoscopic sinus surgery. Am J Rhinol 2005;19:514–20.

[17] Stankiewicz JA, Chow JM. Two faces of orbital hematoma in intranasal (endoscopic) sinus surgery. Otolaryngol Head Neck Surg 1999;120:841–7.

[18] Yung CW, Moorthy RS, Lindley D, et al. Efficacy of lateral canthotomy and cantholysis in orbital hemorrhage. Ophthal Plast Reconstr Surg 1994;10:137–41.

ELSEVIER
SAUNDERS

Otolaryngol Clin N Am
41 (2008) 597–618

OTOLARYNGOLOGIC
CLINICS
OF NORTH AMERICA

Temporal Bone Fracture: Evaluation and Management in the Modern Era

Freedom Johnson, MD[a], Maroun T. Semaan, MD[b],
Cliff A. Megerian, MD, FACS[a],*

[a]*Department of Otolaryngology – Head and Neck Surgery, Case Western Reserve University,
University Hospitals of Cleveland, 11100 Euclid Avenue, Cleveland, OH 44106, USA*
[b]*House Ear Institute, 2100 West 3rd Street, Los Angeles, CA 90057, USA*

Epidemiology and historical background

Approximately 4% to 30% of head injuries involve a fracture of the cranial base, including 18 to 40% with temporal bone involvement [1–4]. Most of these fractures are unilateral, with bilateral fractures reported in 9% to 20% [2,5–7]. These patients frequently present with multiple injuries of varying severity. Although the temporal bone fracture and related sequelae may not represent the patient's most immediately threatening problems, early involvement of the otolaryngologist/neurotologist in evaluation and management can improve long-term functional outcome.

Clinical relevance

The importance of temporal bone fractures relates not only to functional deficits from injury to structures within the temporal bone but also to regional and intracranial complications. The more common sequelae of temporal bone fracture include injury to the facial nerve with facial paresis or paralysis; disturbance of the cochleovestibular apparatus with associated sensorineural hearing loss, conductive hearing loss, balance disturbance, tinnitus, and vertigo; and cerebrospinal fluid (CSF) leak through the fracture lines [1,3,4,6–8]. Less common otologic manifestations include conductive hearing loss secondary to ossicular chain damage, sympathetic sensorineural hearing loss, perilymphatic fistula, posttraumatic endolymphatic hydrops, cholesteatoma, meningocele/encephalocele, and late otogenic meningitis [1,4–6,8–13].

---

* Corresponding author.
E-mail address: cliff.megerian@uhhospitals.org (C.A. Megerian).

0030-6665/08/$ - see front matter © 2008 Elsevier Inc. All rights reserved.
doi:10.1016/j.otc.2008.01.006   *oto.theclinics.com*

Associated injuries to adjacent structures include palsies of other cranial nerves, especially cranial nerves VI and IX through XI, and vascular injury, including carotid artery and sigmoid sinus injuries [5,8,14]. These patients also frequently experience critical intracranial injuries that often dictate their early management, including subarachnoid hemorrhage, subdural hemorrhage, brain contusion, and cerebral edema [3].

Classification systems

Historically, temporal bone fractures have been classified as either transverse or longitudinal based on Ulrich's [15] observations in 1926 and then experiments performed on cadaveric human heads in the 1940s (Figs. 1 and 2) [16]. Based on this initial evidence, and confirmed in clinical series, 80% to 90% of temporal bone fractures are longitudinal and 10% to 20% are transverse [1,16–19].

However, changing patterns of injury over time and the failure of *longitudinal* and *transverse* to accurately describe many clinically observed fractures led to the addition of *oblique* and *mixed* descriptors (Fig. 3) [20]. Despite

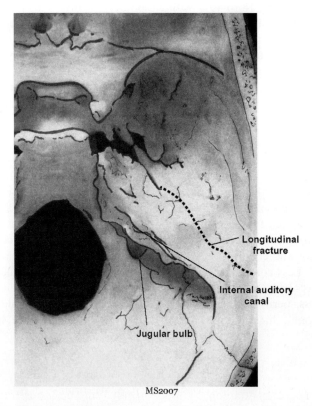

MS2007

Fig. 1. Longitudinal fracture. Note orientation parallel to the long axis of the petrous pyramid.

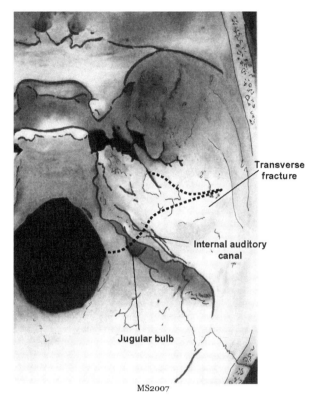

Fig. 2. Transverse fracture. Note orientation perpendicular to the long axis of the petrous pyramid.

improved accuracy in describing the fracture geometry, this expanded terminology still failed to correlate descriptors and clinical sequelae. To address this shortcoming, several authors over the past decade introduced new classification systems in attempt to better correlate fracture geometry with clinical outcomes [7,21,22]. Of these, the classification as otic capsule–violating (OCV) versus otic capsule–sparing (OCS) has been the most predictive of clinical outcome [4,23].

Etiology

The pattern of injuries resulting in temporal bone fracture has evolved over time. With the advent of improved automobile safety technology, the number of fractures from motor vehicle accidents has decreased [1,8]. In contrast, increasing rates of violent crimes have led to increasing rates of temporal bone injury from assault, including those from blunt instruments and firearms [3]. In addition, although overall temporal bone fracture incidence has trended down, advances in pre- and in-hospital trauma care have

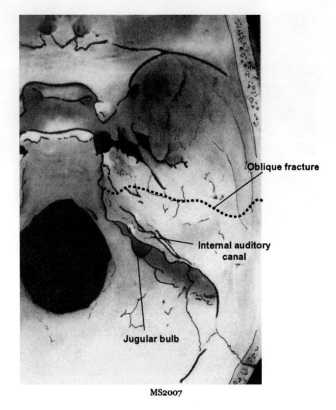

Fig. 3. Oblique fracture. Note the presence of both longitudinal and transverse elements.

led to more patients who have temporal bone fractures surviving their initial injury than previously [24].

In contemporary series, the primary mechanisms of injury include motor vehicle accident (12%–47%), assault (10%–37%), falls (16%–40%), and gunshot wound (3%–33%) [1,3,4,6,7,18,23]. In a subset analysis of 115 patients who had facial paralysis caused by temporal bone fracture, the mechanisms included road traffic (63%), industrial (7%), and sports accidents (3%).

Two unique subpopulations in which these injuries are seen include (1) large urban inner-city hospital settings where blunt assault and gunshot wounds account for most injuries, with a recent trend toward increasing numbers of violence-related temporal bone fractures [3], and (2) the pediatric population that shows a bimodal distribution centered at 3 and 12 years, with falls and motor vehicle accident most prominent in the younger children, and biking accidents and blows to the head more prominent in older children [18,25]. In larger series, children account for 8% to 22% of patients who have temporal bone fracture [1,6]. Of fractures inducing facial paralysis, 9% comprise children, with most injuries being associated with domestic accidents [8].

Anatomic and mechanical factors

Research models

In the 1940s, Gurdjian and Webster [16] extensively studied deformation of the human skull secondary to low-velocity impacts using the "stresscoat" technique. Although they did not have the goal of studying fractures, they showed how force applied to a given point is distributed throughout the cranial skeleton, which led to an understanding of the relationship between point of impact and orientation of fractures.

To study the issue of fracture secondary to automobile accidents, Travis and colleagues [26] conducted a set of experiments on human cadavers involving piston impact to the temporoparietal region and sled tests designed to simulate a side impact automobile accident. In this study, the average force leading to temporal bone fracture was 1875 lb with an average speed of 25 mph. In all cases, this force was enough to produce severe injury to the temporal bone and intracranial contents.

In 2004, Yoganandan and Pintar summarized 150 years of experimental analysis of temporoparietal impact biomechanics. Key findings include [27]:

1. The human head deforms before actual fracture in compression studies.
2. The mechanical properties of the skull do not depreciate significantly with age after maturity, in contrast to other bones such as hips.
3. The temporoparietal region requires as much if not more force to fracture than the frontal region.

Clinical specimen dissections

In 2005, Wysocki [19] conducted a dissection study on 100 temporal bones obtained from forensic autopsy cases. Although the observed fractures and associated injury patterns did not correlate with the mechanism of injury, the study showed the anatomic details of the injury complex as it occurs in real rather than simulated patients. However, possible selection bias must be considered, in that forensics cases may not accurately reflect the pattern of injury in the general population, and many of the specimens originated from cases that did not survive the initial injury and therefore probably represent more severe levels of injury [19].

The detailed analysis showed a fracture pattern of 82% longitudinal, 11% transverse, and 7% mixed, correlating with the reported literature. Injury to the bony facial canal was shown in 44% of bones with longitudinal fractures and 64% of those with transverse fractures. In cases of longitudinal fracture, most facial nerve injuries occurred in the region of the genu, and transection of the nerve was rarely seen. In contrast, in bones with transverse fractures, the nerve injury predominantly occurred in the labyrinthine portion and was usually associated with complete transection of the facial nerve. Ossicular chain injuries consisted of dislocation at the incudomallear joint in 51% and the incudostapedial joint in 57% of patients, malleus fracture in 8%, and stapes fracture in 17%. No bones showed incus fractures. Vascular injuries included injury to the jugular bulb (21%) in association with all fracture orientations, and carotid canal fracture in 52%, although arterial wall injury occurred in only one bone [19].

Radiology

Modalities

Imaging studies play a crucial role in the contemporary evaluation and management of temporal bone fractures. The evaluation of temporal bone fracture requires assessment of not only the temporal bone itself but also the surrounding structures, including the intracranial contents and cervical spine. Before high-resolution CT (HRCT), temporal bone fracture was diagnosed predominately based on clinical grounds. Typical acute clinical indicators of temporal bone fracture include hemorrhagic otorrhea, hemotympanum, tympanic membrane perforation, vertigo, hearing loss, facial nerve palsy, nystagmus, and Battle's sign [1,3,4]. Late indicators include subtle findings of wrinkles or folds in the tympanic membrane or a flaccid tympanic membrane, bony step-offs in the annulus or canal wall, and unexplained hearing loss with a history of head trauma [1].

Noncontrasted HRCT of the temporal bone, with cuts ideally no more than 1.5 mm, is the diagnostic imaging standard for evaluating temporal bone fractures. HRCT provides excellent depiction of bony anatomy (including axial) and reconstructions of coronal and sagittal images from the raw axial data. In addition to delineating fracture anatomy, it also allows evaluation of the facial canal, ossicular chain, otic capsule, carotid canal, and middle cranial fossa floor. Furthermore, contemporary scanners are capable of rapid imaging of critically ill patients with minimal requirements for patient manipulation [28].

Compared with physical examination, HRCT has greater sensitivity. On correlating physical examination findings with HRCT, radiographically evident temporal bone fractures were missed on physical examination in 14% to 35% of patients. This finding has led some authors to recommend HRCT of all patients who have head trauma [3,24].

For evaluating intracranial contents, and for nerve palsy not explained using HRCT, MRI remains the optimal choice once the patient has been stabilized enough to allow for the longer examination time [28]. MRI also plays a role in preoperative evaluation for patients requiring surgical intervention for temporal bone fractures, especially for middle cranial fossa approaches that entail temporal lobe retraction [29]. One series showed a 46% incidence of ipsilateral temporal lobe contusion in patients who needed surgical intervention for facial nerve injury secondary to temporal bone fracture. None of the temporal lobe contusions were clinically evident, and MRI showed four temporal lobe contusions and two subdural hematomas not identified on HRCT [29]. MRI also differentiates between herniation of intra-cranial contents into the mastoid and a fluid-filled mastoid, which frequently cannot be distinguished on HRCT [30].

Additional imaging modalities include traditional four-vessel arteriogra-phy, which remains the gold standard for definitive evaluation of intracra-nial vascular injury, including the temporal portion of the carotid artery, and CT metrizamide cisternography, which can be helpful in localizing otogenic CSF leaks.

Classification systems

The division of temporal bone fractures into longitudinal and transverse has been attributed to Ulrich [15] who described these fracture orientations in 1926. This classification system was reinforced in the 1940s when Gurdjian and Webster used a cadaveric model that supported the classification into longitudinal (80%) and transverse (20%) orientations, and which has been replicated in many clinical series [1,7,16–19]. Longitudinal fractures are described as secondary to temporoparietal impact, leading to fractures exten-ding from the squamosa through the posterosuperior bony external auditory canal, across the tegmen tympani and anterior to the labyrinth, terminating in the middle cranial fossa at the foramen spinosum (see Fig. 1; Fig. 4) [1]. In contrast, transverse fractures result from fronto-occipital blows and course perpendicular to the long axis of the petrous pyramid from the foramen magnum through the posterior fossa, through the petrous pyramid, including the otic capsule, and into the middle cranial fossa (see Fig. 2; Fig. 5) [1].

However, in clinical practice this dichotomous system proved too limiting, with many fractures having mixed components. In some series, up to 62% to 90% of blunt trauma–induced fractures were more accurately described as

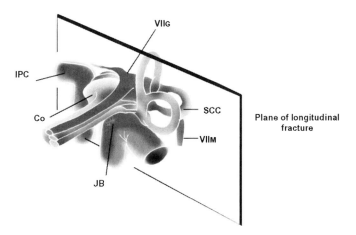

Fig. 4. Plane of longitudinal fracture in relation to the cochleovestibular apparatus. Note the plane passes anterior to the otic capsule.

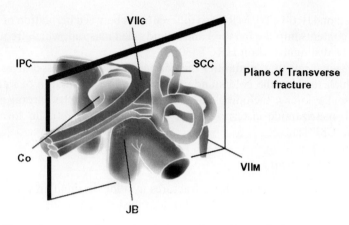

Fig. 5. Plane of transverse fracture in relation to the cochleovestibular apparatus. Note the plane passes through the otic capsule.

mixed [3–5]. In 1992 Ghorayeb and Yeakley [20] proposed the inclusion of the oblique fracture to more accurately describe the three-dimensional anatomy of fracture planes based on the geometry of fractures observed in their series of 150 fractures, with oblique fractures accounting for 75% (see Fig. 3).

Although this classification allowed for more accurate description of fracture patterns, it failed to adequately correlate radiologic findings with clinical outcomes. To address this limitation, Kelly and Tami [21] introduced the concept of OCS versus OCV as descriptors that better correlated with clinical sequelae of temporal bone fracture. In a detailed examination of this system, Dahiya and colleagues [4] found a fourfold increase in CSF leak, a sevenfold increase in sensorineural hearing loss (SNHL) in OCV fractures, and a statistically significant association among OCV fractures, epidural hematoma, and subarachnoid hemorrhage.

Little and Kesser [23] validated these findings, showing a 5-fold increase in facial nerve injury, a 25-fold increase in SNHL, and an 8-fold increase in CSF leak with OCV fractures. They also showed a correlation among OCV fracture and facial nerve paresis or paralysis, conductive hearing loss (CHL), and dizziness or balance dysfunction. In a large series of 820 temporal bone fractures, facial nerve paralysis occurred in 48% of OCV fractures versus only 6% in OCS fractures, and CSF leak occurred twice as frequently in the OCV fractures [6]. In terms of fracture incidence, although some have reported a higher incidence of OVC fractures [23], the incidence is 2.5% to 5.6% in most series [4,6].

More recently, others have introduced a petrous versus nonpetrous fracture classification. Similar to OCS versus OCV, this system groups OCV and petrous apex fractures as "petrous," and fractures involving the middle ear and/or mastoid as "nonpetrous." Using this system, most complications occurred in the petrous group, whereas CHL was uniquely associated with the nonpetrous middle ear fracture group [7]. Validation studies have not yet been reported.

Clinical presentations

Neurologic injury

Because of the tremendous forces required to produce a temporal bone fracture, patients frequently have multiple injuries, with associated nontemporal skull fractures (47%), maxillofacial fractures (21%), and orthopedic injuries outside the head and neck (16%) [3]. Strict adherence to Advanced Trauma Life Support protocols is critical in treating these patients [2].

Many patients present with intracranial injury. In a series of 115 patients with facial paralysis secondary to temporal bone fracture, 33% presented with a Glasgow Coma Scale (GCS) score of less than 7 [8]. In another series, the mean GCS was 12 (range 3–15), with 49% of patients showing mental status changes and 7% having limb paralysis [3]. Despite improved pre- and in-hospital care, mortality related to neurologic sequelae in this population still runs as high as 10% [3,6], and for those who do survive, these severe injuries frequently have significant long-term consequences, with up to 16% of patients requiring institutional care beyond the initial acute management period [3].

Specific intracranial injuries encountered in the temporal bone fracture patient include subdural hematoma (21%), subarachnoid hemorrhage (23%), brain contusion (9%–46%), and tension pneumocephalus [3,29,31]. In a series of 43 patients who had temporal bone fracture, 84% had at least one intracranial pathologic finding, of which 39% had two or more. Overall, 44% of these patients required open neurosurgical intervention, including 86% of those who had two or more findings [3].

Of particular importance in the initial evaluation of patients who have temporal bone fracture is adherence to cervical spine injury precautions. The general rate of cervical spine injury in the blunt trauma setting is 2% to 6% [32]. Although they were not specifically evaluating patients who had temporal bone fracture, Diaz and colleagues [32] reported on cervical spine injury in 1006 patients who had blunt trauma and altered mental status (average GCS of 12). In the setting of altered mental status, cervical spine injury was double the general population at 12%. Of the 116 patients who had cervical spine injuries, 17% had unstable fractures that required further intervention. This study further showed the superiority of HRCT in identifying cervical spine injury, with a missed fracture rate of only 1.7% compared with a miss rate of 52% for plain film radiography [32].

Facial nerve injury

The reported incidence of facial nerve paralysis after temporal bone fracture varies according to fracture pattern. Using the traditional classification system, facial nerve injury occurs in 10% to 25% of longitudinal fractures and 38% to 50% of transverse fractures [2,23]. Brodie and Thompson [6] reported an overall facial nerve injury rate of 7%, correlating with their low incidence of OCV fractures. Facial nerve injury in the pediatric population is much less common, with reports as low as 3%. This finding has been hypothetically attributed to the increased flexibility of the pediatric skull [18].

The timing of onset of facial paralysis has an important bearing on outcome. Immediate paralysis frequently indicates a transection of the nerve with loss of neural continuity, whereas delayed onset paralysis or paresis usually occurs in the context of an intact nerve and denotes the development of neural edema or expanding hematoma with neural compression inside a non-expanding bony canal [8]. Among 7% of patients who had temporal bone fracture with facial paralysis, 27% were immediate onset and 73% were delayed [6]. Darrouzet and colleagues [8] studied 115 patients who had temporal bone fracture with facial nerve injuries and found paresis in 23%, complete immediate paralysis in 52%, complete delayed paralysis in 15%, and 10% whose severe intracranial injuries precluded determination of paralysis onset.

Most injuries occur in the region of the geniculate ganglion or second genu [8,17]. Nerve exploration showed the following lesions: geniculate ganglion in 66%, second genu in 20%, tympanic segment in 8%, and mastoid segment in 6%. Although 91% of patients showed only one injury, geniculate ganglion lesions occurred in conjunction with a separate lesion in the mastoid segment in 6%. The typical pathologic findings included contusion of the nerve, including edema and hematoma of the nerve sheath in 86% and nerve transection, either partial or complete, in 14% of the cases [8]. Other series showed similar findings, with additional notation of fibrosis and bone spicules at the geniculate ganglion in up to 33% of patients [17,33].

Cerebrospinal fluid leak

The reported incidence of CSF leak in temporal bone fracture patients ranges from 11% to 45% [2,6,25]. Most of these represent CSF otorrhea, but in a few cases, an intact tympanic membrane will shunt the fluid to the eustachian tube with resultant CSF rhinorrhea [6,25]. In the acute phase, CSF is often mixed with blood and a high index of suspicion must be maintained for timely diagnosis. The presence of a halo sign, a reservoir sign when patients bend their heads, or clear fluid mixed with dried blood are often suggestive. In cases where the diagnosis is less obvious, fluid can be analyzed for beta-2 transferrin.

The presence of a leak has been correlated with the geometry of the temporal bone fracture with a two- to fourfold increased risk for OCV fractures [4,6]. Brodie and Thompson [6] reported an overall incidence of 18%, of whom 7% developed meningitis. Of these patients, 4% had additional CSF leaks secondary to concurrent anterior basilar skull fractures that also required surgical treatment.Meningitis was much more likely to occur in patients who had a CSF leak lasting more than 7 days and was more prevalent in the pediatric population (4/9 cases; 45%), although they only represented 3% of the study population [6].

Hearing loss

Hearing loss in patients who have temporal bone fracture may be immediate or delayed; may be transient, permanent or progressive; and may have a conductive, sensorineural, or mixed pattern [2,6–8,34]. Reported incidence rates are 26% to 57% for CHL; 14% to 23% for SNHL, including 14% with complete SNHL; and 20% to 55% for mixed [2,5,7,8]. Overall, approximately 24% of patients will have a subjective complaint of hearing loss [6]. In a patient who had known SNHL after bilateral temporal bone fractures, microfractures involving the otic capsule were identified on histopathologic analysis of temporal bones. Although these fractures would escape detection on clinical imaging, these findings may underlie the phenomenon of cochlear concussion, wherein SNHL occurs without gross disruption of the hearing structures [34]. Cochlear concussion was noted in 9% of 115 cases of facial nerve paralysis associated with temporal bone fracture [8]. In an alert patient, a simple tuning fork test may give clues to the nature of the hearing loss. Audiograms are typically performed 3 to 6 weeks after the injury to allow enough time for resolution of hemotympanum, because middle ear fluid (CSF or blood) results in a conductive loss, and behavioral testing after resolution of the fluid will help determine the presence of ossicular discontinuity.

A unique form of delayed hearing loss is progressive SNHL in the contralateral uninjured ear presenting months to years after the initial trauma. Known as *sympathetic hearing loss*, this form of SNHL has a reported incidence of 1% to 11% in patients who have temporal bone fracture [13]. This hearing loss has been shown to be associated with isolated autoimmunity to inner ear antigens [13]. In theory, the cochleovestibular apparatus exists as an immunologically privileged site, and exposure of antigens after trauma is believed to sensitize the general immune system, leading to an autoimmune-mediated contralateral SNHL. Although these patients may initially experience response to steroid treatment, the hearing loss may still progress, in which case excellent response to cochlear implantation has been reported [13].

Other cranial nerve palsies

Depending on the fracture geometry, temporal bone fractures may result in palsies to cranial nerves other than the facial nerve, with a reported incidence of 7.8% [8]. The jugular foramen syndrome consists of palsies of cranial nerves IX, X, and XI and occurs in petrous apex fractures that involve the jugular foramen or its surrounding structures [8,35]. As with the facial nerve, the palsy may be immediate or delayed, with delayed onset portending a better prognosis [35]. Darrouzet and colleagues [8] reported a 2.6% incidence of lower cranial nerve palsy in three cases of jugular foramen hematoma.

Injury to the sixth cranial nerve occurs with an incidence of 5% to 7%, all of which occurred in fractures involving the petrous apex, and including three patients who had bilateral cranial nerve VI palsies associated with bilateral temporal bone fractures [5,8]. This most frequently involves a stretch or impingement injury as the nerve enters Dorello's canal where it passes under the petroclinoid ligament [5]. Although fractures involving this area are likely to lead to a cranial nerve VI injury, this nerve, with its long intracranial course, is subject to stretch injury even in the absence of direct involvement by fracture. This injury is believed to occur during posterosuperior displacement of the brain during impact, causing temporary impingement of cranial nerve VI against the rigid petroclinoid ligament [5]. As a rule, the patient will usually have spontaneous recovery between 2 weeks and 4 months from injury [5,33].

A cranial nerve V palsy has also been reported in a patient who had bilateral temporal bone fractures, bilateral cranial nerve VI palsies, and bilateral cranial nerve VII palsies. The mechanism is believed to be a stretch/impingement injury at the point where the sensory root enters the dural foramen at the entrance of Meckel's cave, which is located just inferior to the margin of the petrous pyramid [5]. Two months after injury and exploration for the cranial nerve VII palsies, the affected trigeminal nerve had regained function [5].

Vascular injury

In an anatomic dissection of 100 temporal bone fractures from autopsy specimens, all injuries involving either the sigmoid groove or the jugular fossa resulted in violation of vessel wall. In contrast, although fractures of the bony carotid canal were common, they rarely disrupted the vessel wall [19]. In a clinical report involving a patient who had bilateral temporal bone fractures, the fracture line extended to the sigmoid sinus, which was found to be thrombosed at exploration for a facial nerve palsy [5]. In this setting of aseptic thrombus, exploration is not usually warranted for the sigmoid sinus thrombus alone, because this region has a rich collateral drainage and therefore presents little threat [5].

With respect to the carotid artery, internal carotid artery dissection with carotido-cavernous fistulae was observed in 1% to 3% of cases [5,8]. Resnick and colleagues [14] examined the relationship between basicranial fracture and carotid artery injury in 230 patients, and found that 55 (24%) patients had fractures involving the carotid canal, 6 (11%) of whom had vascular complications directly related to the intracranial carotid injury. In contrast, only 4 (2.3%) of 175 in the noncarotid canal fracture group sustained vascular complications. Although 62% of fractures occurred at the junction of the lacerum and cavernous portions of the canal, most vascular injuries occurred in fractures of the petrous segment (67% of injuries), with 25% of patients with petrous fractures sustaining a carotid injury [14].

Vertigo

Vertigo frequently occurs after temporal bone trauma and may be secondary to either vestibular concussion in OCS situations or vestibular destruction in OCV settings [1]. The vertigo is usually self-limiting and resolves within 6 to

12 months from central adaptation. Perilymph fistulae can also cause vertigo and may occur with injury to the otic capsule. Although most patients who experience disruption of the otic capsule present with profound SNHL and no vestibular function, some will retain some degree of residual inner ear function. These patients typically present with immediate postinjury fluctuating hearing loss and vestibular symptoms that may persist for months [1,9].

Another cause of vertigo after temporal bone fracture is posttraumatic endolymphatic hydrops. These patients present with aural fullness, tinnitus, fluctuating hearing loss, and vertigo similar to patients who have Meniere's disease [10]. The mechanism is theorized to be a disruption in the endolymph/perilymph balance secondary to an injury to either the membranous labyrinthine duct or the endolymphatic fluid drainage pathways, which occurs in cases of temporal bone fracture through the vestibular aqueduct [10].

Short-term management: days to weeks

Examination

The evaluation and management of any temporal bone fracture patient should include a complete neuro-otologic examination. The examining physician should perform the examination as aseptically as possible. Irrigating the canal is contraindicated, because it may flush contaminated debris into the intracranial space. Likewise, packing the external auditory canal in the setting of suspected CSF otorrhea is contraindicated except in the rare instance of a patient who is exsanguinating, because this will lead to stagnation of fluid and increase the risk for meningitis [1].

Facial nerve injury

The management of facial nerve paralysis depends on the timing of paralysis relative to the injury. Cases involving immediate onset are traditionally managed with surgical exploration after imaging and electrical studies indicate a need for nerve decompression or repair. Cases in which the timing of onset cannot be determined are best considered part of the immediate onset group [6,8]. Patients who have delayed-onset or incomplete paralysis are typically treated with high-dose corticosteroids with further intervention based on results of electrodiagnostic testing or imaging [2,4,8]. Steroid treatment typically begins with 1 mg/kg per day of prednisone or equivalent corticosteroid for 1 to 3 weeks followed by a taper [4,8]. The delay between onset and recovery in spontaneously recovering patients ranges from 1 day to 1 year, with 59% recovery by 1 month and 88% recovery by 3 months [6]. Patients who have delayed-onset paralysis have an excellent prognosis. In two series, 84% to 93% of patients who had delayed-onset paralysis met criteria for conservative treatment. In both series, 100% of these patients recovered to House-Brackmann (HB) grade I or II [4,6].

Further intervention in cases of immediate or uncertain timing of paralysis onset is based on results of electrodiagnostic testing, including electroneuronography and electromyography. Because wallerian degeneration is incomplete in the first 2 weeks after injury, some authors prefer to wait until postinjury day 10 to perform electrodiagnostic testing to improve test reliability [8]. In cases with complete degeneration, testing will often show fibrillation potentials and no response after stimulation. If electroneuronography shows absent responses, electromyography is indicated, because ongoing degeneration and regeneration can cause dyssynchrony of neural input and phase cancellation. In cases of neurapraxia, testing will usually show an absence of voluntary action potentials, but a synchronized evoked response can be observed on nerve stimulation testing [8].

Many authors agree that the threshold for surgical intervention is reached when a 90% or greater degeneration is seen on electroneuronography [2,17], with some investigators reporting this as the key indicator for surgery regardless of timing of paralysis onset [2]. Others base surgical intervention on correlation between electromyography findings and HRCT [8,33] or on documented complete immediate paralysis alone [1,6,8].

Despite earlier reports, nerve exploration has been encouraging in appropriate patients who have facial paralysis related to temporal bone fracture. At 2 years follow-up, 94% to 100% of patients experienced at least a grade III recovery, 45% had a grade I recovery, and no patients had worse than grade IV recovery [8,33]. In another series of 11 operated nerves, 5 recovered to HB I, 4 to HB II, and 2 to HB III [33]. In a subset analysis, 78% of patients who underwent nerve suturing recovered to at least grade III [8].

Advocated surgical approaches vary from transmastoid/supralabyrinthine with conversion to middle cranial fossa if the anatomy is prohibitive, or translabyrinthine in the setting of no serviceable hearing [6,8,17], to primary middle cranial fossa approach in cases of longitudinal fractures and combined middle cranial fossa/transmastoid approach in mixed fracture orientations [8,33].

The goal of complete transection is to repair the nerve in a manner that limits surrounding fibrosis and inflammation and provides rapid and reliable reapproximation of the nerve ends. This goal can be achieved with either primary suture neurorrhaphy or fibrin glue, and can be applied in either end-to-end anastomosis or interposition grafting [36–38]. Using fibrin glue in both primary reapproximation and interposition grafting, Bozorg Grayeli and colleagues [36] achieved an 84% long-term recovery to grade III or better [36]. Fibrin glue has the advantage of technical ease and has acceptable outcomes compared with microsutures with respect to axon regeneration and neurophysiologic properties of the repaired nerve [37,38]. Recovery of facial function after repair is a lengthy process averaging 7 months [36]. A correlation was found between longer duration of nerve interruption and worse outcome after repair [36].

In addition to decompression and repair as appropriate, Darrouzet and colleagues [8] advocate for routine performance of geniculectomy, which they describe as "the removal of the ganglionic contingent lying on the curve of the motor fibers of the VIIth and of the proximal end of the petrous nerves, the distal ends of which are cauterized." The underlying principle is prevention of the crocodile tear syndrome by preventing incorrect regrowth of secretory fibers in the petrous nerves [8].

Cerebrospinal fluid leak

Contemporary management of cerebrospinal fluid leak begins with conservative measures including head elevation, bedrest, stool softeners, avoidance of nose blowing/sneezing and other forms of straining, and, in selected patients, placement of a lumbar drain or intermittent spinal taps [6,25]. In series examining CSF leaks, incidence ranged from 15% to 45% and spontaneous resolution with this conservative management occurred in 95% to 100% of patients [2,4,6,25]. In spontaneously recovering leaks, closure occurred in the first 7 days in 78%, with an additional 17% closing between 8 and 14 days [6].

The role of antibiotic treatment in the setting of CSF leak remains controversial. Brodie and Thompson [6], whose series included 122 patients who had CSF leak, found a meningitis rate of 7% in patients who had CSF leak versus 1% in those who did not. Of patients who had CSF leak who developed meningitis, significant risk factors included leak persisting more than 7 days and the presence of concurrent infection elsewhere. In patients who had CSF leak and concurrent infection, 20% developed meningitis compared with 3% of patients who had CSF leak without concurrent infection. Based on this data, they recommend closure of CSF leaks persisting more than 7 to 10 days but were unable to provide conclusive recommendations on the role of antibiotics [6]. However, in separate meta-analysis, Brodie [39] showed a statistically significant increase in meningitis in patients who had CSF leak who did not receive prophylactic antibiotics.

In the adult and pediatric populations, approximately 5% of patients had CSF leaks persisting beyond 7 to 10 days of conservative therapy and required surgical repair to control the leaks [6,25]. The choice of approach can be directed by preoperative imaging. When HRCT suggests a defect larger than 2 cm, MRI should also be performed to evaluate for potential herniation of intracranial contents into the mastoid/middle ear, and thereby guide the choice of surgical approach [30]. For smaller defects, a transmastoid approach may be adequate; however, larger defects are best approached using an extradural middle cranial fossa approach [6,30].

Hearing loss

Early audiometric evaluation will frequently show CHL secondary to hemotympanum. Nevertheless, this early evaluation is important for documenting a baseline postinjury hearing status, especially relating to SNHL [8]. A subsequent full audiologic workup should be obtained 3 to 6 weeks postinjury to allow enough time for resolution of hemotympanum. This examination will uncover a conductive loss related to ossicular chain disruption and will assess the level of existing SNHL. Vestibular function tests may be helpful in analyzing the vestibular apparatus [1,8,18]. In very young patients who have experienced traumatic brain injury or those who are otherwise uncooperative, auditory brainstem response may be used to obtain a baseline level of auditory function [40].

In the short-term management of CHL, most authors prefer to wait to determine if the loss will resolve spontaneously. However, if earlier neuro-otologic intervention is planned (eg, facial nerve decompression, CSF leak repair), ossiculoplasty can be used as appropriate for concomitant exploration [1,8]. Incidental findings at nerve exploration have included granulations around the ossicles, granulations within the vestibule, and complete fibrous obliteration of the vestibule and semicircular canals [17].

Vertigo

For cases of vertigo secondary to perilymph fistula, preservation of residual auditory and vestibular function and resolution of symptoms have been reported with surgical repair of the fistula, even when performed in a delayed setting [1,9]. Fistulae usually occur at either the oval or round window and may involve subluxation of the stapes footplate, and are typically treated with either patching or obliteration of the niches during middle ear exploration.

Delayed development of posttraumatic perilymphatic hydrops may occur, and patients are usually managed similarly to those who have Meniere's disease. Treatment may include a low-salt diet, steroids, and diuretics. However, the role of endolymphatic shunt surgery has not been systematically investigated in this setting.

Benign paroxysmal positional vertigo (BPPV) is common after trauma and usually develops days to weeks after injury. It is presumably caused by traumatic displacement of otoconia from the vestibule into the ampulla of the posterior semicircular canal. Treatment with standard rehabilitation, including repositioning maneuvers, is usually curative.

Acute unilateral deafferentation caused by ablative injury will usually compensate in a manner and time course similar to acute labyrinthitis or neuronitis.

Other cranial nerve palsies

Patients who have temporal bone fractures may present with palsies of cranial nerves V through XI. As with the facial nerve, some authors advocate early exploration in all case of immediate-onset paralysis. Most would agree with conservative management in cases of delayed onset, because spontaneous recovery is the rule [5,35]. For patients who have cranial nerve VI palsy, some practitioners use patching of the paretic eye. If no recovery occurs by 4 months, then surgical intervention targeted at the affected muscle is indicated [5].

Long-term management: weeks to months

Facial nerve injury

For patients who have persistent facial paralysis after the initial recovery period, late decompression surgery can be beneficial, as shown in seven of nine patients undergoing decompression as late as 3 months who recovered to grade I or II when followed up for at least 1 year [41]. Most patients who have facial paralysis or paresis that does not completely recover in the initial 3 to 4 months are observed for at least 1 year. Preserving eye function is paramount during this time, and attention must be given to proper eye protection with gold weight lid implants or tarsorrhaphy for the nonclosing eye. After 1 year of observation to allow maximal spontaneous recovery, reanimation and reinnervation techniques are usually used [42]. Using the HB grading system, patients who have spontaneous recovery of function at the HB V to VI level are candidates for reinnervation using techniques such as hypoglossal–facial nerve grafts or cross-facial grafting. Because these interventions require another year for development of function, some authors advocate concomitant reanimation with dynamic temporalis slings [43].

Patients who experience recovery to HB III to IV are often offered augmentation procedures, such as brow lift, alar suspension, and botulinum toxin injection for synkinesis. However, no attempt is made to surgically address the facial nerve itself. Patients who experience grade I to II recovery are typically satisfied with their functional and cosmetic outcome and desire no intervention.

Hearing loss

For patients who experience persistent CHL after the acute recuperative 3 to 4 months, ossicular dislocation or fracture must be suspected, and exploration with ossiculoplasty is indicated. The most common finding is incudostapedial dislocation (11%–14%), followed by dislocation of the incudomallear joint [1,5,19]. Additional findings include fracture of the stapes superstructure in 7% and malleus fracture in 1% [1]. In another series, 6 (26%) patients who experienced an initial CHL had a persistent air–bone gap of more than 20 dB. All were explored; five had incudostapedial joint dislocations and one had a stapes fracture, and in all cases the postoperative air–bone gap closed to within 10 dB [2].

Although adults rarely experience fracture of the stapes, children who have persistent CHL after temporal bone trauma have been reported to have an increased incidence of stapes fracture. This finding is theorized to be secondary to the increased deformability of the pediatric skull, and fractures have been noted even in instances associated with minor head trauma [44].

Several therapeutic options exist for treating persistent SNHL. Traditionally, bone-anchored hearing aids have been the best option for auditory rehabilitation in patients who have unilateral profound SNHL, allowing for improved directional discrimination and elimination of the head shadow effect [45]. However, in cases of bilateral severe to profound SNHL, some authors have experienced success with cochlear implantation in appropriately selected patients. Candidates for implantation are patients who have favorable anatomy, including no significant bony discontinuity or cochlear ossification, and for whom promontory testing suggests an intact cranial nerve VIII [46,47]. In a histopathologic study of three patients who had five temporal bone fractures, sufficient neural elements were maintained, even in severe injury, to support the use of cochlear implantation [48]. In a series of seven patients who had temporal bone fracture selected for cochlear implantation, including six who had bilateral temporal bone fractures and one who had preinjury congenital unilateral profound SNHL, all experienced successful rehabilitation. Two of the seven experienced stimulation of the facial nerve, which could not be programmed out. This condition was believed to be secondary to an electrical leak through fractures lines, and explantation with contralateral implantation yielded good results [46]. Patients who have mild to moderate SNHL are usually treated with standard amplification.

Posttraumatic endolymphatic hydrops–related hearing loss

Given the infrequent occurrence of endolymphatic hydrops in the setting of temporal bone fracture, few authors have addressed its treatment. Drawing on experience with patients who had Meniere's disease, a similar initial treatment approach seems reasonable. If patients remain symptomatic after a trial involving diuretics and a low-sodium diet, then surgical exploration may be considered, primarily to address the possibility of an undiagnosed perilymphatic fistula. However, no data support the use of endolymphatic sac decompression and shunt in this setting.

Management of delayed sequelae: years to decades

Meningocele/encephalocele

A meningocele and an encephalocele are rare late phenomena that can present with delayed onset of CSF otorrhea, unilateral clear middle ear effusion, or recurrent meningitis. Reported presentations range from 1 to 21 years after initial trauma [49]. Given the late presentation and nonspecific symptom complex, delayed diagnosis frequently occurs. These conditions often present after clear otorrhea is discovered when tubes are placed to equalize pressure for presumed serous otitis media. These delayed-onset herniations should be approached in the same manner as those that are more immediate, including combined transmastoid/middle cranial fossa approaches for large defects (> 1 cm) or transmastoid approach alone for smaller defects [49].

Cholesteatoma

Cholesteatoma represents another rare late complication, with fewer than 20 reported cases [12]. Presentations occurred 2 to 24 years after injury. Cholesteatomas are frequently extensive, and may present as otogenic brain abscesses; one patient even presented 2 years after sustaining a temporal bone fracture with symptoms including a 5-day history of fever, otalgia, vomiting, and headache, and a 3-month history of personality changes. This patient developed a large temporoparietal brain abscess that was successfully treated with neurosurgical drainage followed by a canal wall down tympanomastoidectomy [12]. At mastoidectomy he was found to have a cholesteatoma arising from the posterosuperior aspect of the bony external auditory canal [12]. McKennan and colleagues [50] reported on three patients who developed cholesteatoma 3 to 7 years postinjury, two who had no prior intervention and one who underwent previous transmastoid/middle fossa facial nerve exploration. The authors theorized on an etiology of traumatic implantation of epithelial elements at injury, and postulated that the more extensive growth frequently noted in comparison with other cholesteatomas occurs because posttraumatic cholesteatomas usually arise in the setting of a well-pneumatized adult temporal bone [50]. McGuirt and Stoole [25] noted two patients in the pediatric population who had cholesteatoma. One occurred in the fracture line of a conservatively treated fracture, and the other in an obliterated fracture. In an interesting subset, 2 of 13 (15%) patients surviving gunshot wounds to the temporal bone subsequently required mastoidectomy for secondary cholesteatoma [6].

Late cerebrospinal fluid leak

Late CSF leak may occur spontaneously or in the setting of meningocele/encephalocele or cholesteatoma. In the latter situations, treatment should be provided in the manner discussed earlier. In cases of spontaneous CSF leak, a search for the leak must be undertaken and the defect repaired, as with early nonspontaneously resolving CSF leaks.

Late meningitis

Patients who have fractures violating the otic capsule have been noted to have an increased long-term risk for meningitis. This trend is believed to occur because the enchondral bone of the otic capsule heals through a fibrous rather than osseous process [6,11]. This complication can be a life-threatening, as shown by a case report of a patient who developed an acute otitis media years after a temporal bone fracture. This acute otitis ultimately progressed to a lethal meningitis. Histopathologic analysis of the patient's temporal bone showed an acute purulent labyrinthitis in the old fracture line that was filled with fibrous tissue and extended into the internal auditory canal [11]. To prevent further episodes, these cases should be treated with a labyrinthectomy and fat graft obliteration with closure of the external auditory canal.

Summary

Temporal bone fractures rarely occur in isolation. The comprehensive evaluation and management of patients who have temporal bone fracture frequently requires cooperation among trauma surgeons, radiologists, neurosurgeons, and otolaryngologists and neurotologists. Early management focuses on stabilization of the patient, with subsequent efforts focused on treating facial paralysis, CSF leak, and hearing impairments. The late occurrence of potentially life-threatening complications, including meningitis, cholesteatoma, and herniation of intracranial contents through the skull base, mandates long-term close follow-up of these patients with early attention to any signs of potential late sequelae.

References

[1] Cannon CR, Jahrsdoerfer RA. Temporal bone fractures. Review of 90 cases. Arch Otolaryngol 1983;109(5):285–8.
[2] Nosan DK, Benecke JE Jr, Murr AH. Current perspective on temporal bone trauma. Otolaryngol Head Neck Surg 1997;117(1):67–71.
[3] Alvi A, Bereliani A. Acute intracranial complications of temporal bone trauma. Otolaryngol Head Neck Surg 1998;119(6):609–13.
[4] Dahiya R, Keller JD, Litofsky NS, et al. Temporal bone fractures: otic capsule sparing versus otic capsule violating clinical and radiographic considerations. J Trauma 1999; 47(6):1079–83.
[5] Ghorayeb BY, Yeakley JW, Hall JW 3rd, et al. Unusual complications of temporal bone fractures. Arch Otolaryngol Head Neck Surg 1987;113(7):749–53.
[6] Brodie HA, Thompson TC. Management of complications from 820 temporal bone fractures. Am J Otol 1997;18(2):188–97.
[7] Ishman SL, Friedland DR. Temporal bone fractures: traditional classification and clinical relevance. Laryngoscope 2004;114(10):1734–41.
[8] Darrouzet V, Duclos JY, Liguoro D, et al. Management of facial paralysis resulting from temporal bone fractures: our experience in 115 cases. Otolaryngol Head Neck Surg 2001; 125(1):77–84.
[9] Lyos AT, Marsh MA, Jenkins HA, et al. Progressive hearing loss after transverse temporal bone fracture. Arch Otolaryngol Head Neck Surg 1995;121(7):795–9.
[10] Shea JJ Jr, Ge X, Orchik DJ. Traumatic endolymphatic hydrops. Am J Otol 1995;16(2): 235–40.
[11] Sudhoff H, Linthicum FH Jr. Temporal bone fracture and latent meningitis: temporal bone histopathology study of the month. Otol Neurotol 2003;24(3):521–2.
[12] Majmundar K, Shaw T, Sismanis A. Traumatic cholesteatoma presenting as a brain abscess: a case report. Otol Neurotol 2005;26(1):65–7.
[13] ten Cate WJ, Bachor E. Autoimmune-mediated sympathetic hearing loss: a case report. Otol Neurotol 2005;26(2):161–5.

[14] Resnick DK, Subach BR, Marion DW. The significance of carotid canal involvement in basilar cranial fracture. Neurosurgery 1997;40(6):1177–81.

[15] Ulrich K. Verletzungen des Gohororgans bei Schadelbasisfrakturen. (Eine histologische und klinisshe Studie). Acta Otolaryngol Suppl 1926;6:1–150.

[16] Gurdjian ES, Webster JE. Deformation of the skull in head injury studied by stresscoat technique. Surg Gynecol Obstet 1946;83:219–33.

[17] Coker NJ, Kendall KA, Jenkins HA, et al. Traumatic intratemporal facial nerve injury: management rationale for preservation of function. Otolaryngol Head Neck Surg 1987; 97(3):262–9.

[18] Lee D, Honrado C, Har-El G, et al. Pediatric temporal bone fractures. Laryngoscope 1998; 108(6):816–21.

[19] Wysocki J. Cadaveric dissections based on observations of injuries to the temporal bone structures following head trauma. Skull Base 2005;15(2):99–106.

[20] Ghorayeb BY, Yeakley JW. Temporal bone fractures: longitudinal or oblique? The case for oblique temporal bone fractures. Laryngoscope 1992;102(2):129–34.

[21] Kelly KE, Tami TA. Temporal bone and skull trauma. In: Jackler RK, Brackmann DE, editors. Neurotology. St. Louis (MO): Mosby; 1994. p. 340–60.

[22] Yanagihara N, Murakami S, Nishihara S. Temporal bone fractures inducing facial nerve paralysis: a new classification and its clinical significance. Ear Nose Throat J 1997;76(2): 79–80, 83–6.

[23] Little SC, Kesser BW. Radiographic classification of temporal bone fractures: clinical predictability using a new system. Arch Otolaryngol Head Neck Surg 2006;132(12):1300–4.

[24] Exadaktylos AK, Sclabas GM, Nuyens M, et al. The clinical correlation of temporal bone fractures and spiral computed tomographic scan: a prospective and consecutive study at a level I trauma center. J Trauma 2003;55(4):704–6.

[25] McGuirt WF Jr, Stool SE. Cerebrospinal fluid fistula: the identification and management in pediatric temporal bone fractures. Laryngoscope 1995;105(4 Pt 1):359–64.

[26] Travis LW, Stalnaker RL, Melvin JW. Impact trauma of the human temporal bone. J Trauma 1977;17(10):761–6.

[27] Yoganandan N, Pintar FA. Biomechanics of temporo-parietal skull fracture. Clin Biomech (Bristol, Avon) 2004;19(3):225–39.

[28] Schuknecht B, Graetz K. Radiologic assessment of maxillofacial, mandibular, and skull base trauma. Eur Radiol 2005;15(3):560–8.

[29] Jones RM, Rothman MI, Gray WC, et al. Temporal lobe injury in temporal bone fractures. Arch Otolaryngol Head Neck Surg 2000;126(2):131–5.

[30] Nishiike S, Miyao Y, Gouda S, et al. Brain herniation into the middle ear following temporal bone fracture. Acta Otolaryngol 2005;125(8):902–5.

[31] Kuncz A, Roos A, Lujber L, et al. Traumatic prepontine tension pneumocephalus—case report. Ideggyogy Sz 2004;57(9–10):313–5.

[32] Diaz JJ Jr, Gillman C, Morris JA Jr, et al. Are five-view plain films of the cervical spine unreliable? A prospective evaluation in blunt trauma patients with altered mental status. J Trauma 2003;55(4):658–63.

[33] Ulug T, Arif Ulubil S. Management of facial paralysis in temporal bone fractures: a prospective study analyzing 11 operated fractures. Am J Otolaryngol 2005;26(4):230–8.

[34] Ohlrogge M, Francis HW. Temporal bone fracture. Otol Neurotol 2004;25(2):195–6.

[35] Yildirim A, Gurelik M, Gumus C, et al. Fracture of skull base with delayed multiple cranial nerve palsies. Pediatr Emerg Care 2005;21(7):440–2.

[36] Bozorg Grayeli A, Mosnier I, Julien N, et al. Long-term functional outcome in facial nerve graft by fibrin glue in the temporal bone and cerebellopontine angle. Eur Arch Otorhinolaryngol 2005;262(5):404–7, Epub 2004 Sep 15.

[37] Ornelas L, Padilla L, Di Silvio M, et al. Fibrin glue: an alternative technique for nerve coaptation—Part I. Wave amplitude, conduction velocity, and plantar-length factors. J Reconstr Microsurg 2006;22(2):119–22.

[38] Ornelas L, Padilla L, Di Silvio M, et al. Fibrin glue: an alternative technique for nerve coaptation—Part II. Nerve regeneration and histomorphometric assessment. J Reconstr Microsurg 2006;22(2):123–8.

[39] Brodie HA. Prophylactic antibiotics for posttraumatic cerebrospinal fluid fistulae. A meta-analysis. Arch Otolaryngol Head Neck Surg 1997;123(7):749–52.

[40] Lew HL, Lee EH, Miyoshi Y, et al. Brainstem auditory-evoked potentials as an objective tool for evaluating hearing dysfunction in traumatic brain injury. Am J Phys Med Rehabil 2004;83(3):210–5.

[41] Quaranta A, Campobasso G, Piazza F, et al. Facial nerve paralysis in temporal bone fractures: outcomes after late decompression surgery. Acta Otolaryngol 2001;121(5):652–5.

[42] Cheney ML, Megerian MA, McKenna MJ. Rehabilitation of the paralyzed face. In: Cheney ML, editor. Facial surgery: plastic and reconstructive. Baltimore (MD): Williams & Wilkins; 1997. p. 655–85.

[43] Cheney ML, McKenna MJ, Megerian CA, et al. Early temporalis muscle transposition for the management of facial paralysis. Laryngoscope 1995;105(9 Pt 1):993–1000.

[44] Singh S, Salib RJ, Oates J. Traumatic fracture of the stapes suprastructure following minor head injury. J Laryngol Otol 2002;116(6):457–9.

[45] Baguley DM, Bird J, Humphriss RL, et al. The evidence base for the application of contralateral bone anchored hearing aids in acquired unilateral sensorineural hearing loss in adults. Clin Otolaryngol 2006;31:6–14.

[46] Camilleri AE, Toner JG, Howarth KL, et al. Cochlear implantation following temporal bone fracture. J Laryngol Otol 1999;113(5):454–7.

[47] Simons JP, Whitaker ME, Hirsch BE. Cochlear implantation in a patient with bilateral temporal bone fractures. Otolaryngol Head Neck Surg 2005;132(5):809–11.

[48] Morgan WE, Coker NJ, Jenkins HA. Histopathology of temporal bone fractures: implications for cochlear implantation. Laryngoscope 1994;104(4):426–32.

[49] Souliere CR Jr, Langman AW. Combined mastoid/middle cranial fossa repair of temporal bone encephalocele. Skull Base Surg 1998;8(4):185–9.

[50] McKennan KX, Chole RA. Post-traumatic cholesteatoma. Laryngoscope 1989;99(8 Pt 1): 779–82.

ELSEVIER
SAUNDERS

Otolaryngol Clin N Am
41 (2008) 619–632

OTOLARYNGOLOGIC
CLINICS
OF NORTH AMERICA

Facial Nerve Paralysis

Christopher J. Danner, MD

*Tampa Bay Hearing and Balance Center, Otology/Neurotology/Skull Base Surgery,
Harbourside Medical Tower, 4 Columbia Drive, Suite 610, Tampa, FL 33606, USA*

Emotions are communicated through facial expression. Happiness, confusion, and frustration can be expressed with a slight smile, eyebrow shift, or wrinkled nose. Injury to the facial nerve and subsequent inability of perform volitional mimetic movement can provoke anxiety [1]. This article explores the causes, treatment, and prevention of facial nerve paralysis.

Overview

The facial nerve traverses a bony canal in the temporal bone as it courses from the brainstem to the face and neck. The narrowest portion of this canal is the meatal segment, which is located at the transition zone between the lateral portion of the internal auditory canal and the proximal fallopian canal (Fig. 1). Depending on the extent of injury sustained, the facial nerve will lose function in a graduated fashion. If edema is minimal, the nerve will be anatomically intact and a conduction blockade (neuropraxia) will be the only result, and the nerve will recover function quickly and fully without deficit. As nerve injury increases so do sequela from the injury [2]. As the edema increases, the nutrients to the nerve diminish as axoplasmic flow decreases. This decrease in flow ultimately results in axonal death (axonotmesis) [3]. The axon will degenerate in a retrograde fashion to the narrowest portion of the facial canal. With this type of injury, the endoneurium is intact and the axon will regrow through the undisturbed axonal channels, resulting in normal facial function. Any increased injury at this point will result in disruption of the endoneurium (neurotmesis), allowing the regenerating axons to regrow haphazardly. Depending on the extent of nerve disruption this haphazard growth will lead to a variable degree of synkinesis [4].

As a general rule, all patients who have facial paralysis should undergo imaging studies to evaluate the course of the nerve from the brain through

E-mail address: cdanner@tampabayhearing.com

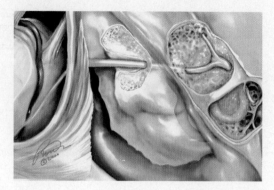

Fig. 1. Middle fossa exposure of the internal auditory canal and tympanic portions of the facial nerve. (*From* Danner CJ, Dornhoffer JL, Linskey M. Facial nerve. In: Sekhar LN, Fessler RG, editors. Atlas of neurosurgical techniques: brain. New York: Thieme; 2006. p. 882–4; with permission.)

the parotid. This evaluation is best performed with a thin-cut contrasted MRI through the temporal bone and upper neck. Patients who have facial paralysis secondary to trauma should undergo a thin-cut temporal bone CT scan [5,6].

Bell's palsy

Rapidly progressive facial paralysis over 24 or 48 hours is most likely secondary to idiopathic nerve edema. The nerve edema is believed to be caused by a viral insult from either activation of a latent herpetic infection or a newly acquired upper respiratory track virus. Bell's palsy is differentiated from other causes of facial paralysis by the absence of trauma and its rapid onset over several hours. This history of rapid progression helps differentiate it from facial paralysis secondary to tumor involvement, which progresses slowly over weeks to months.

Facial paralysis secondary to viral insult is usually self-limited. Depending on the extent of the nerve edema, recovery occurs within days to weeks but can take several months in severe cases. Initiating steroids early (prednisone, 1 mg/kg, for 1 week with a taper) can minimize progressive edema, diminishing further nerve damage and speeding recovery. Studies have shown mixed results on the efficacy of empiric use of antiviral medication. However, valacyclovir was recently associated with earlier recovery and better long-term facial nerve function [7].

Patients who have observable facial movement with an incomplete paralysis experience uniformly good recovery. Recovery may be prolonged and incomplete for patients who have a dense House-Brackmann 6 paralysis (Table 1). Some authors advocate decompressing the facial nerve if facial nerve degeneration is rapid and severe [8]. Although literature supports

Table 1
House-Brackmann facial nerve paralysis classification

Class	General	Symmetry at rest	Synkinesis	Movement	Eye closure
1	Normal	Yes	No	Normal	Yes
2	Slight Weakness	Yes	No	Weak	Yes
3	Can close eye	Yes	Yes	Weak	Yes
4	Cannot close eye	Yes	Yes	Weak	No
5	Slight movement	No	Yes	Slight	No
6	Paralyzed	No	N/A	No	No

Abbreviation: N/A, not applicable.

facial nerve decompression for severe cases of Bell's palsy, the recovery rate remains good without surgical intervention and most surgeons reserve decompression for patients who have recurrent paralysis.

Iatrogenic

Iatrogenic trauma to the facial nerve should be addressed as soon as the injury is recognized. Optimal choices for reconstruction depend on the site of injury and the length of nerve involved.

Unintentional iatrogenic facial nerve paralysis is traumatic for patients and physicians. Operating surgeons often should obtain a second opinion from an experienced physician who can offer an unemotional objective assessment of the severity of injury and propose appropriate treatment options [9–11].

Fortunately, one of the more common causes of unintentional iatrogenic facial nerve paralysis is overzealous use of local anesthetic. In an attempt to obtain adequate anesthesia, particularly for surgical cases performed primarily using local anesthesia, physicians may be tempted to use more anesthetic than they would otherwise. The anesthetic may track along the stylomastoid suture line and anesthetize the facial nerve at the stylomastoid foramen. When facial nerve injury is not expected and a patient experiences immediate postoperative paralysis, physicians may want to wait a few hours to allow the effects of the local anesthetic to wear off before deciding whether further intervention is needed. Frequently, facial function will begin returning within an hour if lidocaine was used, or longer if Marcaine was used. Once adequate time is allowed for the effects of local anesthesia to dissipate and the patient continues to show complete facial paralysis, the facial nerve should be identified and its course followed to locate the site of injury [12].

For patients who have undergone otologic surgery, the facial nerve should be identified at the proximal tympanic segment as it courses from the geniculate ganglion superior to the cochleariform process, and followed to the pyramidal turn down to the stylomastoid foramen (Fig. 2). All areas along the course of the intratemporal facial nerve are potential sites of

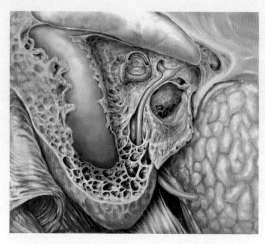

Fig. 2. Transmastoid exposure of descending portion of facial nerve. (*From* Danner CJ, Dornhoffer JL, Linskey M. Facial nerve. In: Sekhar LN, Fessler RG, editors. Atlas of Neurosurgical Techniques: Brain. New York: Thieme; 2006. p. 882–4; with permission.)

injury. When dissecting cholesteatoma in the epitympanum and supratubal recess, the geniculate ganglion and proximal tympanic segment of the facial nerve are at risk for injury [13]. The cochleariform process, which is the exit site of the tensor tympani tendon, is an excellent landmark for the tympanic portion of the facial nerve as it passes just superior to it. The pyramidal turn is another vulnerable site as the nerve turns from its course under the horizontal semicircular canal and descends through the mastoid to the stylomastoid foramen [14]. A blood vessel supplying the nerve in this area is often present to warn the surgeon that the nerve is near by [15].

The descending or mastoid portion of the nerve can also be injured. A common practice for identifying the facial nerve is to open the mastoid air cells, identify the horizontal semicircular canal, and follow the digastric ridge to the stylomastoid foramen and then thin the external auditory canal in a stepwise fashion, working lateral to medial between the landmarks of the stylomastoid foramen and the horizontal semicircular canal. The descending portion of the facial nerve tracks laterally as it progresses to the stylomastoid foramen and may be lateral to the tympanic ring inferiorly [16]. This important anatomic relationship is important when performing a canaloplasty. The facial nerve is vulnerable to injury when expanding the canal in a posterior inferior direction (see Fig. 2).

Once the site of nerve injury is identified, if disruption to the nerve is 50% or less than the total cross-sectional area, then adequate function should return and it is best to leave the nerve alone to minimize any further damage. If more than 50% is traumatized, then the injured portion of the nerve should be removed and an end-to-end anastomosis performed [17]. It is important that a tension-free anastomosis is performed. Tension increases the amount of fibrotic in growth and subsequently decreases the number of axons that are able to propagate distally. If extra nerve length is needed, then the fallopian canal should be opened from the cochleariform process to the stylomastoid foramen. The nerve can then be rerouted directly from these two landmarks, thereby straightening the pyramidal turn and gaining approximately 1 cm in length to perform a tension-free end-to-end anastomosis [18].

If the length of nerve damage is greater than can be compensated for by rerouting, a nerve graft should be used. Many potential sites are available to harvest nerve for a cable graft, but the most commonly used are the great auricular nerve and the sural nerve.

Temporal bone fracture

Fractures of the temporal bone are typically comminuted and vary tremendously depending on the mechanism of injury. Despite the variability that occurs with temporal bone fractures, they can generally be categorized into two groups based on the location of the major fracture lines and how they relate to the axis of the petrous pyramid. When the fracture line is parallel to the posterior petrous face, it is categorized as a longitudinal fracture; when it runs perpendicular across the posterior petrous face, it is a transverse fracture. Most significant facial nerve injury, caused by nonpenetrating temporal bone trauma, occur in the perigeniculate area as a consequence of traction injury from the greater superficial petrosal nerve (GSPN) (Fig. 3) [19–23].

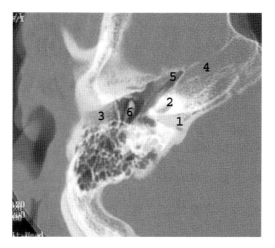

Fig. 3. Axial CT of right temporal bone (several images are combined to show anatomy at several levels). (1) Internal auditory canal. (2) Basal turn of cochlear. (3) External auditory canal. (4) Internal carotid artery. (5) Eustachian tube. (6) Malleus–incus complex.

Longitudinal temporal bone fracture

The area of impact is typically to the temporoparietal skull and results in a longitudinal fracture that courses along the superior external auditory canal into the middle ear and then travels along the eustachian tube and carotid canal to the foramen lacerum (Fig. 4). Because of the location of this fracture line, the tympanic membrane and ossicular chain are usually disrupted, with associated conductive hearing loss and bloody otorrhea. Facial nerve paralysis can occur with longitudinal temporal bone fractures because of traction injury caused to the geniculate ganglion by the GSPN. Furthermore, with severe ossicular disruption, the body of the incus may be displaced sufficiently to traumatize the tympanic portion of the facial nerve. Longitudinal fractures make up approximately 80% of temporal bone fractures. Because the location of the fracture lines typically parallel the facial nerve, they cause facial nerve injury only 20% of the time. For partial facial weakness, a watch-and-wait approach should be used. If facial paralysis is determined to be complete and immediate at the time of injury, an evoked electromyographic recording should be obtained of the facial nerve. When the nerve has degraded more than 90% in less than 2 weeks from the time of injury and no voluntary motor unit potentials are present, surgical decompression of the facial nerve should be considered [22–26].

Transverse temporal bone fracture

Impact typically occurs in the occipital area of the skull. Transverse fractures run perpendicular to the posterior petrous face as they course from the foramen magnum to the foramen ovale. Because these fractures are perpendicular to the axis of the petrous pyramid, they often traverse the otic

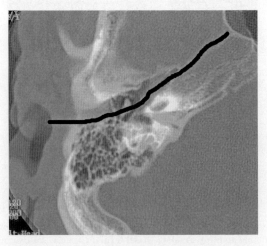

Fig. 4. Location of longitudinal temporal bone fracture.

capsule, causing sensory hearing loss and vertigo. These fractures also typ-ically cross the fallopian canal, causing facial nerve injury (Fig. 5). Although transverse fractures are uncommon, accounting for only 20% of temporal bone fractures, they are responsible for facial nerve injuries 50% of the time. The fracture line frequently does not involve the tympanic membrane or ear canal, and therefore the ear canal is often dry with no signs of otor-rhea. The tympanic membrane is often intact with an associated hemotym-panum. The approach for treatment and decompression is the same as for longitudinal fracture [23,25,26].

Penetrating trauma

Because of the protective effects of the temporal bone, injury to the facial nerve from penetrating trauma typically occurs extracranially. Penetrating trauma resulting in facial nerve injury can be classified as either a proximal or distal nerve injury, depending on the relationship to the lateral canthus of the eye. When injury is medial to the lateral canthus of the eye, usually only the midface facial branches are injured and patients recover nicely without nerve exploration. When injury occurs lateral to the canthus, multiple branches may be involved, substantially affecting upper and lower facial function. Facial nerve dissection and reanastomosis are recommended for proximal nerve injuries within 3 days of the injury. During this time the dis-tal nerve branches can still be stimulated electrically, aiding in their location. When nerve injury occurs at the stylomastoid foramen a mastoidectomy should be performed and mastoid tip removed in order to expose an ade-quate portion of the facial nerve proximal to the site of injury. This allows easy identification of the proximal and distal nerve stumps [27].

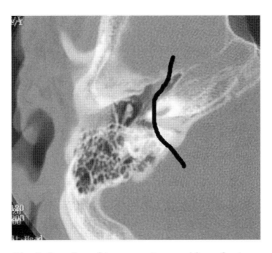

Fig. 5. Location of transverse temporal bone fracture.

Treatment

Medical

Incomplete paralysis caused by nonpenetrating trauma has an excellent prognosis and can be managed expectantly. Penetrating trauma that globally affects the nerve may also be managed expectantly if movement is noted. Regardless of mechanism of injury, steroids are recommended soon after injury to minimize nerve edema and degradation in nerve function from decreased axoplasmic flow (prednisone, 1 mg/kg, for 7 days followed by taper). Because the nerve lies within a bony canal, edema will cause a depression in nerve function. Recent articles have shown a potential benefit from valacyclovir in the treatment of Bell's palsy. If complete facial paralysis (no movement noted in any branch with maximal voluntary effort) occurs after injury, the nerve should be evaluated with electromyography to test volitional and evoked responses. If nerve function degrades 90% or more within the first 2 weeks of injury, then the patient may benefit from surgical decompression. It is important to wait at least three days from the time of injury before obtaining an electromyographic (EMG) study of the facial nerve. If an EMG is performed too early it will give erroneously good results.

Surgical

Decompression

If within 2 weeks from injury facial nerve function degrades to less than 10% of normal then facial nerve function may be improved through surgical decompression. Immediately after injury the distal portion of the facial nerve is still healthy and easily stimulated even with complete nerve transection. Electromyographic analysis of the nerve must not occur until at least 3 days after injury to allow sufficient time for wallerian degeneration to occur. This will allow the health of the facial nerve distal to the injury can be more accurately represented. When more than 90% of the nerve function has degraded, decompressing the facial nerve within 2 weeks from onset of complete paralysis has been shown to improve overall outcome [28].

The narrowest portion of the facial nerve is at the meatus along the proximal labyrinthine portion. If the surgeon decides to decompress the facial nerve, the labyrinthine portion should be decompressed. Access to this portion of the facial nerve can be achieved through a middle fossa craniotomy if the hearing is intact, or through the translabyrinthine approach if hearing is absent [29].

Anastomosis

When the facial nerve is transected or sufficiently injured, requiring the injured portion to be removed, a tension-free end-to-end anastomosis is the best option to reestablish nerve integrity. The facial nerve can be rerouted in the middle ear and 1 cm of additional length can be achieved

[30]. To reroute the facial nerve, it is dissected out of the fallopian canal and is routed directly from the geniculate ganglion, which lies just above the cochleariform process, to the stylomastoid foramen. To achieve proper, safe nerve dissection and anastomosis, it is often wise to take the canal wall down, remove the tympanic membrane and external auditory canal skin, and oversew the ear canal. This procedure allows good visualization and adequate space to perform the anastomosis while also providing adequate protection afterward.

When performing the anastomosis, the nerve ends should be prepared, cleaning extraneous fibrous tissue that may inadvertently fall between the anastomotic ends. A fresh scalpel blade should be used to freshen the nerve to minimize crush injury [31]. A small monofilament suture (8-0 or smaller) with a tapered needle should be used. The sutures should be placed in the peripheral epineurium to minimize injury to individual nerve fascicles (Fig. 6). As few sutures as possible should be placed to achieve an even co-aptation of the nerve ends [32].

When additional nerve length is needed, an intervening nerve graft is used.

Cable graft

Final facial nerve function is worse with a cable graft than a single end-to-end anastomosis because the newly growing axons have two anastomoses to traverse instead of one [33].

Donor sites

Great auricular nerve

One landmark for finding the great auricular nerve is halfway between the mastoid tip and angle of the mandible. A perpendicular line is drawn

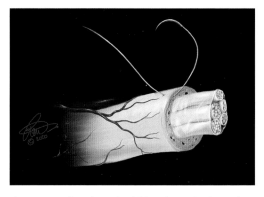

Fig. 6. Before suturing nerve, epineurium should be trimmed. Figure shows proper placement of suture through trimmed epineurium. (*From* Danner CJ, Dornhoffer JL, Linskey M. Facial nerve. In: Sekhar LN, Fessler RG, editors. Atlas of Neurosurgical Techniques: Brain. New York: Thieme; 2006. p. 882–4; with permission.)

in this area and roughly correlates to the location of the nerve. A second landmark is midway along the sternocleidomastoid muscle. The great auricular
nerve emerges along the posterior side of the sternocleidomastoid roughly
halfway between the mastoid tip and the medial clavicular head. Using these
two landmarks, one can reliably locate the nerve for a potential graft (Fig. 7).
The great auricular nerve can provide a maximal length of 10 cm for reconstruction. When longer length is needed, the sural nerve is used.

Sural nerve

Although the diameter is similar to the facial nerve, the sural nerve is often the second choice after the great auricular graft secondary to its unfavor-
able branching pattern and inconvenient location. When using the sural
nerve for a facial nerve graft, the nerve should be reversed before making
the anastomosis. This technique allows the neurons of the facial nerve to
grow in a retrograde fashion along the newly grafted sural nerve and prevents the developing facial nerve tendrils from erroneously traversing the
dead-end paths of the branches originating from the main trunk. To keep
the nerve properly oriented, a suture is placed on the proximal portion of
the nerve before it is removed from the harvest site. This sutured end will
become the distal end of the graft in the recipient bed [34].

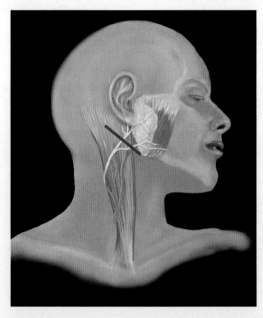

Fig. 7. The great auricular nerve is located halfway between the mastoid tip and angle of the
mandible. (*From* Danner CJ, Dornhoffer JL, Linskey M. Facial nerve. In: Sekhar LN, Fessler
RG, editors. Atlas of Neurosurgical Techniques: Brain. New York: Thieme; 2006. p. 882–4;
with permission.)

The sural nerve has a consistent location. It courses along the lateral lower leg just behind the lateral malleolus and runs parallel to the lesser saphenous vein. A straightforward way to find the sural nerve is to make a small incision immediately posterior to the lateral malleolus and first identify the lesser saphenous vein. The sural nerve can then be found running parallel to this vein and can be traced as it courses superiorly toward the knee (Fig. 8). The sural nerve can provide up to 35 cm of length for cable grafting.

Hypoglossal facial

If the proximal facial nerve is unavailable for grafting, a jump graft is the next best option to provide innervation to the facial mimetic muscles [35]. The hypoglossal is the preferred nerve in jump nerve grafts because it is a strong nerve that not only gives facial symmetry at rest but can also provide mimetic facial movement through training. Its cortical representation is also similar to the facial nerve, making mimetic movements easier to perform. The anastomosis may be performed through sacrificing the hypoglossal nerve and performing an end-to-end anastomosis with the facial nerve or performing an end-to-side anastomosis [36]. The end-to-end anastomosis sacrifices the hypoglossal nerve, causing tongue atrophy and mild articulation difficulties, but is associated with stronger facial movements. The end-to-side anastomosis preserves some tongue function, although the tongue tends to be weak [37]. This weakness is easily compensated for but may not be desirable if the patient already has multiple cranial nerve palsies.

The hypoglossal nerve is found immediately inferior to the posterior belly of the digastric muscle. The nerve traverses the upper neck just superior to

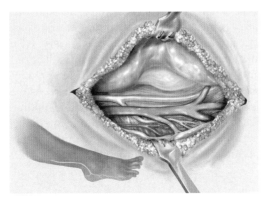

Fig. 8. Location of sural nerve, posterior to lateral malleolus and follows course of lesser saphenous vein. (*From* Danner CJ, Dornhoffer JL, Linskey M. Facial nerve. In: Sekhar LN, Fessler RG, editors. Atlas of Neurosurgical Techniques: Brain. New York: Thieme; 2006. p. 882–4; with permission.)

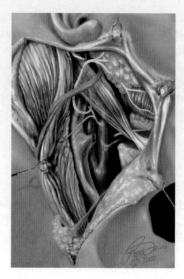

Fig. 9. Hypoglossal facial nerve anastomosis. Hypoglossal nerve is cut distal along its course to give additional length. (*From* Danner CJ, Dornhoffer JL, Linskey M. Facial nerve. In: Sekhar LN, Fessler RG, editors. Atlas of Neurosurgical Techniques: Brain. New York: Thieme; 2006. p. 882–4; with permission.)

the posterior cornu of the hyoid bone and exits the skull base medial to the internal jugular vein. The hypoglossal nerve runs lateral to the external carotid artery and is tethered inferiorly in the angle created by the occipital artery as it exits the posterior side of the external carotid artery (Fig. 9) [38].

Eye care

Regardless of the extent of facial nerve injury, the surgeon must ensure that the eye is adequately protected. Even with minor injuries, blink reflexes can be diminished, increasing the likelihood of corneal injury. Also, if any traction injury is present along the GSPN, the parasympathetic fibers innervating the lacrimal gland may be damaged, which will cause a dry eye and increase the likelihood of corneal ulceration. Patients should use lubricating drops throughout the day and apply hydrating ophthalmic ointment in the evening before bed. Patients should also be followed up by an ophthalmologist until facial function returns. Upper-lid gold weights and canthopexies may also be considered for patients who have anticipated long-term facial weakness.

References

[1] Coulson SE, O'Dwyer NJ, Adams RD, et al. Expression of emotion and quality of life after facial nerve paralysis. Otol Neurotol 2004;25(6):1014–9.

[2] Pillsbury HC 3rd. Pathophysiology of facial nerve disorders. Am J Otol 1989;10(5):405–12.

[3] Selesnick SH, Patwardhan A. Acute facial paralysis: evaluation and early management. Am J Otolaryngol 1994;15(6):387–408.

[4] Moran LB, Graeber MB. The facial nerve axotomy model. Brain Res Brain Res Rev 2004; 44(2–3):154–78.

[5] Roob G, Fazekas F, Hartung HP. Peripheral facial palsy: etiology, diagnosis and treatment. Eur Neurol 1999;41(1):3–9.

[6] Haberkamp TJ, Harvey SA, Daniels DL. The use of gadolinium-enhanced magnetic resonance imaging to determine lesion site in traumatic facial paralysis. Laryngoscope 1990; 100(12):1294–300.

[7] Gilden D, Tyler K. Bell's palsy–is glucocorticoid treatment enough? N Engl J Med 2007; 357(16):1653–5.

[8] Gantz BJ, Rubinstein JT, Gidley P, et al. Surgical management of Bell's palsy. Laryngoscope 1999;109(8):1177–88.

[9] Fenton JE, Fagan PA. Iatrogenic facial nerve injury. Laryngoscope 1995;105(4 Pt 1):444–5.

[10] Schuring AG. Iatrogenic facial nerve injury. Am J Otol 1988;9(5):432–3.

[11] Wiet RJ. Iatrogenic facial paralysis. Otolaryngol Clin North Am 1982;15(4):773–80.

[12] Green JD Jr, Shelton C, Brackmann DE. Iatrogenic facial nerve injury during otologic surgery. Laryngoscope 1994;104(8 Pt 1):922–6.

[13] Eftekharian A. Facial nerve in middle ear and mastoid surgery. Otol Neurotol 2005;26(5): 1093 [author reply: 1093].

[14] Selesnick SH, Lynn-Macrae AG. The incidence of facial nerve dehiscence at surgery for cholesteatoma. Otol Neurotol 2001;22(2):129–32.

[15] Nilssen EL, Wormald PJ. Facial nerve palsy in mastoid surgery. J Laryngol Otol 1997; 111(2):113–6.

[16] Adad B, Rasgon BM, Ackerson L. Relationship of the facial nerve to the tympanic annulus: a direct anatomic examination. Laryngoscope 1999;109(8):1189–92.

[17] Green JD Jr, Shelton C, Brackmann DE. Surgical management of iatrogenic facial nerve injuries. Otolaryngol Head Neck Surg 1994;111(5):606–10.

[18] Dew LA, Shelton C. Iatrogenic facial nerve injury: prevalence and predisposing factors. Ear Nose Throat J 1996;75(11):724–9.

[19] Ishman SL, Friedland DR. Temporal bone fractures: traditional classification and clinical relevance. Laryngoscope 2004;114(10):1734–41.

[20] Yeoh TL, Mahmud R, Saim L. Surgical intervention in traumatic facial nerve paralysis. Med J Malaysia 2003;58(3):432–6.

[21] Adkins WY, Osguthorpe JD. Management of trauma of the facial nerve. Otolaryngol Clin North Am 1991;24(3):587–611.

[22] Adegbite AB, Khan MI, Tan L. Predicting recovery of facial nerve function following injury from a basilar skull fracture. J Neurosurg 1991;75(5):759–62.

[23] Fisch U. Prognostic value of electrical tests in acute facial paralysis. Am J Otol 1984;5(6): 494–8.

[24] Chang C, Cass S. Management of facial nerve injury due to temporal bone trauma. Am J Otol 1999;20(1):96–114.

[25] Barrs DM. Facial nerve trauma: optimal timing for repair. Laryngoscope 1991;101(8): 835–48.

[26] Stennert E. Indications for facial nerve surgery. Adv Otorhinolaryngol 1984;34: 214–26.

[27] May M, Sobol SM, Mester SJ. Managing segmental facial nerve injuries by surgical repair. Laryngoscope 1990;100(10 Pt 1):1062–7.

[28] Marais J, Murray JA. Repair of the injured facial nerve. Clin Otolaryngol Allied Sci 1995; 20(5):387–9.

[29] Myckatyn TM, Mackinnon SE. The surgical management of facial nerve injury. Clin Plast Surg 2003;30(2):307–18.

[30] Piza-Katzer H, Balogh B, Muzika-Herczeg E, et al. Secondary end-to-end repair of extensive facial nerve defects: surgical technique and postoperative functional results. Head Neck 2004;26(9):770–7.

[31] Spector JG. Neural repair in facial paralysis: clinical and experimental studies. Eur Arch Otorhinolaryngol 1997;254(Suppl 1):S68–75.

[32] Gardetto A, Kovacs P, Piegger J, et al. Direct coaptation of extensive facial nerve defects after removal of the superficial part of the parotid gland: an anatomic study. Head Neck 2002;24(12):1047–53.

[33] Meyer RA. Nerve harvesting procedures. Atlas Oral Maxillofac Surg Clin North Am 2001; 9(2):77–91.

[34] Choi D, Dunn LT. Facial nerve repair and regeneration: an overview of basic principles for neurosurgeons. Acta Neurochir (Wien) 2001;143(2):107–14.

[35] Danner CJ, Dornhoffer JL, Linskey ME. Cranial nerve seven reconstruction. In: Sekhar L, Fessler R, editors. Atlas of neurosurgical techniques. New York: Thieme; 2007. p. 882–4.

[36] Rebol J, Milojkovic V, Didanovic V. Side-to-end hypoglossal-facial anastomosis via transposition of the intratemporal facial nerve. Acta Neurochir (Wien) 2006;148(6):653–7 [discussion: 657].

[37] Atlas MD, Lowinger DS. A new technique for hypoglossal-facial nerve repair. Laryngoscope 1997;107(7):984–91.

[38] Asaoka K, Sawamura Y, Nagashima M, et al. Surgical anatomy for direct hypoglossal-facial nerve side-to-end "anastomosis". J Neurosurg 1999;91(2):268–75.

ELSEVIER
SAUNDERS

Otolaryngol Clin N Am
41 (2008) 633–649

OTOLARYNGOLOGIC
CLINICS
OF NORTH AMERICA

Sudden Hearing Loss

Matthew R. O'Malley, MD, David S. Haynes, MD*

*The Otology Group Vanderbilt, 300 20th Ave N., Suite 502, Nashville,
TN 37203-2115, USA*

Sudden sensorineural hearing loss has been described as a medical emergency in search of appropriate diagnostic techniques and treatments [1]. The abrupt development of an unexpected sudden sensory deficit warrants consideration of this situation as an emergency by medical professionals and lay personnel. Despite the dramatic presentation, in most cases, sudden sensorineural hearing loss is the presenting symptom of a pathophysiology that has yet to be identified. In as many as 88% of patients, a battery of diagnostic testing fails to yield an identifiable cause [2].

Sudden sensorineural hearing loss is an active topic of discussion and research in the otolaryngology literature. Over the past 30 years, greater than 800 articles, or roughly one every 2 weeks, has been published on this topic in the English medical literature. Several excellent broad-based reviews of this topic have been written by respected clinicians [1–6], and courses on this subject are regularly presented at professional meetings.

The incidence of sudden hearing loss in the United States is often reported at between 5 and 20 cases per 100,000 people annually, based on a report by Byl [7]. Another commonly quoted figure is that there are roughly 4000 cases annually in the United States [8]. These numbers seem discrepant because 4000 cases annually calculates to 1.3 cases per 100,000 people per year in the United States, currently with a population of roughly 300 million people [9]. Even using the lowest end of Byl's estimate produces 15,000 cases per year in the United States. A recent 5-year study in Thailand demonstrated the incidence to range from 6.49 to 10.21 cases per 100,000 per year, with an average of roughly 8 cases per 100,000 population per year [10].

In its most nonspecific interpretation, the term *sudden hearing loss* could conceivably refer to any sudden loss of hearing (ie, sudden sensorineural hearing loss or sudden conductive hearing loss). Despite this, the term *sudden hearing loss*, and the abbreviation SHL in reference to sudden

---
* Corresponding author.
E-mail address: david.haynes@vanderbilt.edu (D.S. Haynes).

0030-6665/08/$ - see front matter © 2008 Elsevier Inc. All rights reserved.
doi:10.1016/j.otc.2008.01.009   *oto.theclinics.com*

sensorineural hearing loss is frequently found in the literature [5]. Sudden sensorineural hearing loss is also abbreviated as SSHL and sometimes referred to as sudden deafness [8]. For the purposes of this article, sudden hearing loss (SHL) refers to sudden sensorineural hearing loss. The National Institute on Deafness and Other Communication Disorders (NIDCD) [8] defines sudden sensorineural hearing loss as a rapid loss of hearing, occurring over a period of up to 3 days. The hearing loss must be of at least 30 dB in three connected frequencies. Further, the NIDCD indicates that sudden sensorineural hearing loss should be considered a medical emergency, although other investigators openly dispute this [11].

The definition of SHL as a minimum of 30 dB loss over three consecutive frequencies occurring in fewer than 3 days is not universally adhered to in the literature [6]. Some studies do not provide a specific definition for SHL [12,13], whereas others use alternate definitions (such as a 20-dB loss) [14]. The use of unclear or alternate definitions for SHL produces substantial difficulty in comparing patient populations and treatment outcomes among studies; however, there are some justifiable reasons for using an alternate definition of SHL. For example, the sudden development of a 25-dB hearing loss at three consecutive octaves in the range of human speech would likely be noticed and distressing to a normally hearing individual, yet the definition of SHL suggests that a 25-dB loss should not be considered pathologic. Further, in the authors' experience, the presentation of a patient who reports truly progressive loss over 3 days is far less common than presentation of an abrupt loss of hearing marked by a specific point in time. It seems reasonable to propose that rapidly progressing hearing loss may be a different disease entity than hearing loss that occurs at a definable time point. Presumably, these reasons for using an alternate definition of SHL may be considered by some investigators who include patients who have lesser degrees of hearing loss or more rapid progression of symptoms in studies of SHL.

In addition, modern reports tend to treat the term SHL as a diagnosis and thus limit the report or study to only those patients who have idiopathic SHL. Older reports of SHL may be more likely to consider SHL as a symptom and thus include patients in whom the diagnostic evaluation reveals an obvious cause (eg, an acoustic neuroma). Although not all investigators adhere rigorously to the definition espoused by the NIDCD, most studies include patients who have suffered at least a loss of 20 dB at more than one frequency over less than a 72-hour period.

Regardless of how one defines SHL, there is some agreement that the natural course of those who suffer idiopathic SHL involves a spontaneous recovery of function in a percentage of patients. Although the natural course of disease has not been established in a large number of patients, spontaneous recovery is variably reported to occur in up to 65% of patients who have idiopathic SHL [3]. Although the percentage of patients experiencing spontaneous recovery varies in different series, two of the larger series involving patients followed without treatment reported spontaneous recovery rates of 58% (n = 52) [3] and 65% (n = 28) [15].

The likelihood that future studies will include large numbers of untreated patients is small. Various forms of treatment have become widely accepted as beneficial in most locations, and the idea of not providing such treatments could possibly be viewed as unethical. Typically, much of the recovery is thought of as occurring within the first month after the SHL event; however, a recent report found that nearly 22% of patients showed improvement in their audiometric studies beyond the first month following the onset of symptoms [16].

The specific definition of what constitutes "improvement" or "recovery" after an SHL is not uniform among studies and reports. Vague subcategories of recovery, such as partial recovery or minimal recovery, are presented in the literature without universally accepted definitions. Perhaps the most lenient and possibly the most commonly encountered definition of improvement is an improvement of 10 dB in pure-tone average (PTA) or an improvement of 10% or 15% in speech discrimination score (SDS). An alternate, stricter interpretation is improvement of 20 dB in PTA or 20% in SDS. Further, some investigators use a mathematic formula to calculate recovery as a percentage of hearing recovered [17]. Each of these definitions has advantages and disadvantages. Using absolute values of improvement has the advantages of being relatively simple and being able to be performed without knowledge of prior hearing function or a normally hearing contralateral ear. The disadvantage is that absolute values can be misleading in certain patients. For example a patient who has a 90-dB PTA and a 10% SDS could be considered improved at an 80-dB PTA and a 10% SDS, even though the patient may not notice any subjective improvement. Further, patients who experience improvement in PTA but a worsening SDS (or vice versa) may be classified as improved. Presenting recovery as a percentage is more complex but provides consideration for a varying spectrum of severity of sudden loss. A major disadvantage to presenting recovery as a percentage is the need to know or assume the function of the ear before the SHL event. In most cases, an audiogram before the SHL event is not available and must be assumed. Typically, the ear is assumed to be normal or similar to the contralateral ear. The validity of these assumptions has an impact on the calculation of a recovery percentage.

Most important, the lack of a uniform definition of recovery limits the ability to compare or combine data across studies. In a recent article, the authors and colleagues [18] presented data using four different definitions of recovery to compare their data to those of other studies. The recovery rates between their study and three other studies were found to be reasonably similar when identical definitions were applied. It seems reasonable to speculate that perhaps the applied definition of recovery is the single most important factor in determining what percentage of patients who have SHL recover.

Beyond the differing definitions of SHL and the dispute over how to best evaluate the presence or absence of recovery from a sudden loss, several important questions regarding sudden sensorineural hearing loss remain unanswered. The cause of SHL remains obscure in most cases. The role and value of diagnostic testing is uncertain and, thus, the evaluation of patients presenting with SHL is not standardized. Perhaps most pertinent to its consideration as an emergency is this question: Is there any treatment that provides better patient outcomes than simply observing the natural course of the disease?

Etiology

The list of agents linked to the development of SHL ranges from snake venom to oral contraceptives [4]. Some of these agents may legitimately cause SHL, whereas others are likely the result of simple association. Box 1 presents a list of some causes associated with the development of SHL. Some conditions such as vestibular schwannoma are known to present with SHL and can be readily diagnosed with an appropriate evaluation. SHL in most patients, however, has no identifiable cause. A review of 837 patients diagnosed with SHL between 1989 and 1993 found that 88% were ultimately deemed idiopathic [2].

Although the list of potential etiologies is lengthy, the more substantial evidence seems to support that idiopathic SHL is most commonly the result of viral infection, vascular disruption, or an autoimmune processes. None of these etiologies has undisputed evidence supporting its role in the cause of SHL; therefore, these cases remain idiopathic. Reviews on the potential etiologies of SHL are readily available [4,19,20].

The concept that a viral infection can cause SHL seems reasonably well supported. Congenital infection with certain viral agents (cytomegalovirus, rubella, herpesvirus) is associated with hearing loss [19]. Viral labyrinthitis induced in animals can create a reversible SHL [21]. Epidemiologic evidence has linked a specific viral illness (Lassa fever) to SHL [22,23]. There is a strong reason to suspect that viral infections can affect the facial nerve and vestibular nerve, causing acute facial palsy or vestibular neuronitis. These entities bear striking similarity to SHL, in that they begin suddenly, often without warning, and spontaneous recovery of function is seen in a variable percentage of patients. A similar process could occur in the cochlear nerve, causing potentially reversible hearing loss.

Similar to the concept that viral infection may cause SHL, the concept of vascular disruption is also reasonably well supported. Ischemic events affecting the auditory pathway have been demonstrated in some patients who have SHL [24]. Certain prothrombotic risk factors and genes have been associated with SHL [25,26]. Plasmapheresis and other treatments designed to alter blood viscosity have been reported to help recovery [27].

Box 1. Causes associated with development of hearing loss

Infectious causes
Meningitis (streptococcal, meningococcal, cryptococcal)
Mumps
Rubeola
Rubella
Syphillis
Herpesvirus (simplex, zoster, varicella)
Lassa fever
HIV/AIDS
Mononucleosis
Mycoplasma
Toxoplasmosis
Cytomegalovirus

Toxic causes
Snake bite
Ototoxic agents

Immunologic causes
Wegener's granulomatosis
Cogan's syndrome
Primary immune inner ear disease

Other causes
Meniere's disease
Hyperostosis cranialis interna
Pseudohypoacusis

Neoplastic causes
Acoustic neuroma
Meningioma
Lymphoma
Leukemia
Myeloma
Meningeal carcinomatosis

Neurologic causes
Multiple sclerosis
Neurosarcoidosis

Circulatory causes
Cerebrovascular accident
Sickle cell disease
Cardiopulmonary bypass
Vertebrobasilar insufficiency

Traumatic causes
Temporal bone fracture
Acoustic trauma
Barotrauma
Perilymph fistula
Otologic surgery

The idea that hearing loss may be the result of an autoimmune process is attributed to McCabe [28]. Subsequent studies have supported this premise, and specific autoantibodies have been identified and proposed to cause hearing loss [29]. Further, the association of SHL with known autoimmune diseases such as Cogan's syndrome, Wegener's granulomatosis, and temporal arteritis has been well documented [30].

All of these proposed etiologies seem reasonable; however, they all have significant flaws when applied broadly to all cases of SHL. After much discussion, many investigators might concede that SHL likely represents the common symptom of a number of different pathologies, but on the whole, it is not known what causes most cases of SHL.

Lastly, one should carefully consider cochlear membrane rupture as a cause of SHL. Practical clinical experience with temporal bone trauma, stapedectomy surgery, and other aspects of common otology has shown that damage to the internal membranes of the cochlea can result in hearing loss. Thus, in the appropriate clinical setting, accepting cochlear membrane rupture as an etiology for SHL seems appropriate. The concept of spontaneous cochlear membrane rupture is different. Unlike the notion that SHL may be caused by viral, vascular, or autoimmune causes, there seems to be little objective evidence to support the idea that a substantial percentage of idiopathic SHL is caused by a spontaneous cochlear membrane rupture.

Evaluation

Evaluation of patients who have SHL varies substantially among clinicians. Overtly, the goal of the evaluation should be to detect known causes of SHL. To this end, the evaluation should begin with history taking. The main elements of the history include the time of onset, progression or fluctuation since onset, and the presence or absence of any other noticed neurologic deficits. The presence of vestibular symptoms, tinnitus, or a feeling of aural fullness should be elicited and may suggest onset of Meniere's disease. Diagnostic criteria for this disorder are readily available [31]. The presence of aural pain may be seen with infectious causes; however, a few patients report pain in the presence of a normal examination. In older reports, the history of an antecedent upper respiratory tract infection was often reported and thought to possibly correlate with a viral cause of SHL. Although this approach seems logical, an informal evaluation of this concept by Mattox and Simmons [3] found that roughly 25% of patients who had SHL reported an anteceded upper respiratory tract infection, which was very similar to a control population.

The patient should be questioned about trauma to the ear and about the presence of autoimmune diseases in the patient or family members. A history of sexually transmitted disease exposure should be reviewed in an attempt to screen for neurosyphilis. Exposure to ototoxic agents should be explored. Travel to exotic locations may suggest etiologies that are less often encountered by the treating physician. A surprising number of patients report that the hearing loss was noticed immediately on awakening, suggesting that the hearing loss occurred during sleep; the significance of this is not known.

One particularly unresolved area of evaluation involves Lyme disease. Lyme disease has been associated with the development of SHL and with the development of other cranial neuropathies, including facial paralysis [32,33]. It is tempting to ask the patient about previous tick bites and possibly obtain Lyme titers in an attempt to evaluate the patient for zoonotic causes for SHL. Any such evaluation should be undertaken with caution, however, because a percentage of the asymptomatic population is positive for Lyme titers, and the incidence and prevalence of the disease can vary dramatically in different geographic areas. Beyond these diagnostic difficulties, the appropriate treatment for those who have SHL associated with Lyme disease is disputed. The input of an infectious disease specialist or neurologist who has a particular interest in Lyme disease may be appropriate in patients in whom this diagnosis seems pertinent. At present, there does not seem to be satisfactory evidence in the literature with which to resolve this issue.

Although not generally useful for diagnostic purposes, the duration of time from the onset of symptoms until presentation at the otolaryngologist's office may be one of the most important factors in determining a patient's prognosis. Most patients do not seek treatment immediately at the onset of symptoms, and the typical presentation is generally delayed 48 to 96 hours. As is discussed later, substantial evidence that treatment rendered by the otolaryngologist is primarily responsible for an improvement in outcome over the natural course of the disease is not in abundance. Thus, it has been suggested that a certain percentage of patients who develop symptoms have spontaneous improvement within a few days of onset and are less likely to present for evaluation. Patients whose symptoms last beyond a few days are more likely to present for evaluation, and these patients may be less likely to improve [3].

Many studies acknowledge that some degree of vertigo or imbalance is present in a percentage of patients who have SHL [2,3]. The criteria distinguishing SHL with vertigo from acute labyrinthitis are not formally defined. To a rough approximation, it seems that a patient who presents due to hearing loss and acknowledges a mild degree of imbalance is more likely to be diagnosed with SHL, and a patient who presents with a chief complaint of vertigo and is found to have hearing loss is more likely to be diagnosed with labyrinthitis. The use of objective tests of vestibular function to distinguish the two diagnoses does not appear to be commonplace.

The physical examination of the patient who has SHL should include a standard otolaryngologic examination, with specific attention to known causes of SHL. A neurotologic examination with otoscopic examination to evaluate for effusion, infection, and certain neoplasms is essential, along with thorough evaluation of the cranial nerves and cerebellar function. The nasal septum should be examined for evidence of autoimmune processes.

Following the history and physical examination, the audiometric evaluation should be reviewed. For the purposes of comparison, the audiometric evaluation should include PTA (0.25 kHz, 0.5 kHz, 1 kHz, 2 kHz, 4 kHz [or 3 kHz], and 8 kHz) and SDS to evaluate severity of initial loss and the degree of recovery.

In most instances, MRI of the brain and internal auditory canals enhanced with gadolinium contrast should be obtained in most patients to identify treatable, serious causes of sudden loss (eg, acoustic neuroma, cerebrovascular accident). For patients in whom MRI scanning is contraindicated, a contrasted CT scan of the head with thin cuts may be an appropriate substitute and should be able to identify larger lesions. Consultation with a neuroradiologist may allow such a CT scan to be optimized to detect smaller lesions.

Beyond the previously described measures, the evaluation of patients who have SHL is extremely variable from one clinician to another. Laboratory evaluations including complete blood count, basic or complete metabolic panels, electrolyte levels, and sedimentation rate are undoubtedly reasonable, although many clinicians no longer obtain these studies routinely because the diagnostic yield is low. Rheumatologic workup including sedimentation rate and antinuclear antibodies are indicated when the history is suggestive of autoimmune causes. Fluorescent treponemal antibody testing may be appropriate when suspicion for neurosyphilis is high, although some investigators have pointed out that the false-positive rate in an otologic population may be high [34]. Large panels of viral titers seem to have been largely abandoned, although selected titers may be appropriate based on the clinician's impression. Laboratory testing of vestibular dysfunction is generally not necessary for patients who have SHL. Patients who have balance complaints significant enough to warrant objective testing may often be relegated to an alternate diagnosis.

Management

The management of SHL is perhaps the most controversial aspect of this entity. The medical literature contains seemingly innumerable reports touting various treatment agents and regimens. The use of more than one agent in treatment is exceedingly common, and the choice of agents used varies substantially among clinicians. In the United States, oral steroids remain the mainstay of treatment. Certain other treatments are commonly employed and enjoy relatively widespread support; specifically, transtympanic steroids perfusions and oral antiviral agents. The use of treatments such as carbogen gas inhalation, hyperbaric oxygen treatment, diuretics, plasma expanders, and agents designed to alter blood flow or viscosity is not unusual, although these agents are perhaps less commonly employed in the current environment. In regions outside the United States, other therapies enjoy much wider acceptance. For example, in central Europe, hypervolemic hemodilution is one of the more commonly employed treatment regimens [35]. To date, no treatment agent or scheme is universally accepted, and no single agent has been irrefutably determined to improve or worsen patient outcomes beyond the natural history of the disease. A partial list of treatments advocated in the literature is presented in Box 2.

Oral steroids

In 1980, Wilson and colleagues [15] presented the results of a double-blind placebo-controlled trial evaluating the efficacy of steroids in treating SHL. Most saliently, the study found an improvement rate of 61% for those treated with steroids compared with 32% for those treated with placebo. This demonstration of efficacy has, at least in part, been responsible for the widespread implementation of oral steroids as treatment for SHL in the United States. A few important aspects of this study bear mentioning. First, in addition to the treatment and placebo groups, there was a third group of patients— untreated control subjects (presumably patients who did not receive placebo or steroids)—who showed a recovery rate almost identical to those treated with steroids (58%). Second, two clinical sites contributed patients to the study. The steroid regimens were not the same at the two clinical sites: patients at one site were treated with 10 days of dexamethasone starting at 4.5 mg twice daily, whereas those at the second site were treated with 12 days of methylprednisolone starting at 16 mg, three times daily.

Within recent years, several investigators have reported their own refinements to the treatment of SHL with oral steroids. Slattery and colleagues [36] presented a review from the House Ear Institute in 2006 that found that optimal results were achieved with a 14-day prednisone taper, starting at 60 mg orally daily. Others have advocated more aggressive regimens. Narozny and colleagues [37] presented a group of patients treated with 1000 mg methylprednisolone intravenously for 3 days combined with an oral prednisone taper starting at 60 mg daily and found that this treatment combined with other treatments produced improved outcomes compared with other regimens tried at their center.

Other studies fail to confirm the efficacy of oral steroids in treating SHL [38,39]. A randomized double-blind placebo-controlled trial presented in 2001 found that 60% of those who took oral steroids improved compared with 63% of those who received a placebo [38]. Further, the association of worse clinical outcomes with increasing steroid doses has been reported in a retrospective review of 250 patients [39]; thus, the concept that oral steroids are to be universally accepted as a benign, yet potentially helpful intervention, that can cause no morbidity, is challenged.

Several well-written reviews of the use of oral steroids in the treatment of SHL have been presented [40–42]. A 2006 Cochrane database review concluded that the value of steroids in the treatment of SHL remains unclear [40]. Conlin and Parnes [41,42] similarly concluded that no valid randomized

Box 2. Sensorineural hearing loss treatments

Oral steroids
   Prednisone
   Dexamethasone
   Methylprednisolone
   Betamethasone
Transtympanic steroids
   Dexamethasone
   Methylprednisolone
Intravenous steroids
   Methylprednisolone
Oral antivirals
   Acyclovir
   Valacyclovir
Hemodilution
   Dextran
   Hydroxyethyl starch
Vasodilators
   Histamine
   Papaverine
   Verapamil
   Procaine hydrochloride
   Cyclandelate
Carbogen gas inhalation
Hyperbaric oxygen therapy
Vitamins
   B_1
   B_3
   B_6
   B_{12}
   E
Diuretics
   Mannitol, others
Antibiotics
Magnesium
Betahistine
Pentoxifylline
Vinpocetine
Thrombolytics
   Tissue plasminogen activator
   Batroxibin
Anticoagulants

Sodium enoxaparin
Heparin
Plasmapheresis
Stellate ganglion block
Dorsal sympathectomy
Benzodiazepenes
Interferon-α
ATP
Diatrizoate meglumine (Hypaque)
Xanthinolnictone
Probanthine
Ginkgo biloba
Lipoprostaglandin E_1
Intravenous lidocaine
Repeated smallpox vaccination
Dietary/lifestyle modifications
  Restriction of caffeine
  Cessation of smoking

controlled trial exists to determine effective treatment of SHL, and that systemic steroid use cannot be considered the gold standard of treatment for SHL. Despite these systematic reviews, clinicians practicing in the United States are cautioned to consider offering steroids to those who present with SHL because certain practitioners and publications may consider this treatment to represent a gold standard in treatment.

Transtympanic steroids

Transtympanic steroid injection (also called intratympanic steroid perfusion) was applied to the treatment of Meniere's disease in 1991 [43]. Based on the acceptance of systemic steroid therapy for treatment of SHL, the use transtympanic steroids for the treatment of SHL was proposed by Silverstein and colleagues [44] in 1996. Animal studies conducted by Parnes and colleagues [45] and Chandrasekhar [46] demonstrated that transtympanic steroid perfusion results in dramatically higher concentrations of steroids in the labyrinth. Based on these studies and on favorable initial clinical evaluations, clinicians have embraced transtympanic steroid perfusion as a treatment modality. The advantages and disadvantages of transtympanic steroid administration compared with systemic steroid administration are presented in Box 3.

The use of intratympanic steroids has evolved into three main protocols for treatment of sudden SHL: (1) initial or primary treatment for sudden SHL without systemic steroids, (2) adjunctive treatment given concomitantly

---

Box 3. Transtympanic steroids

Advantages
Assured compliance
May be suitable for patients in whom systemic steroids
   are contraindicated or declined
Therapy directed to the affected ear
Higher concentration of steroids in the ear
Few side effects, complications
Office-based procedure, accomplished without general
   anesthetic
Well tolerated

Disadvantages/complications
Pain
Tympanic membrane perforation
Otitis media
Vertigo (usually temporary)
Hearing loss

---

with systemic steroids for sudden SHL, and (3) "salvage therapy" after failure of systemic steroids for sudden SHL.

Beyond these three general protocols, there is substantial diversity among clinicians with regard to the type and amount of steroid used and the timing and frequency of administration.

A number of investigators have presented series of patients who have SHL treated with transtympanic steroids [18,45–50]. Most of these studies are retrospective reviews of clinical experience and none have definitively established the efficacy of transtympanic steroids as superior to the natural rate of recovery. A large multicenter trial is underway to better resolve this issue, and results are expected within the next few years.

Oral antiviral agents

The use of antiviral agents to treat SHL is relatively widespread. Contemporary literature suggests that most practitioners are using oral antiviral agents; however, the use of intravenous agents, including interferon, has been reported [51]. Oral antiviral agents have been described as potentially beneficial [52]. Two randomized double-blind placebo-controlled trials have been conducted, one evaluating valacyclovir [53] and the other evaluating acyclovir [54]. Both studies failed to show significant improvement with the use of an oral antiviral agent. Despite these negative trials, oral antiviral agents remain commonly employed in the treatment of SHL, and not without reason. Animal studies have shown that animals that have herpes simplex virus labyrinthitis treated with acyclovir combined with pred-nisolone suffer less cochlear damage than animals treated with either agent alone [21]. If one assumes that a small minority of patients suffer SHL due to a viral infection caused by a virus susceptible to acyclovir or valacyclovir, and that treatment of patients with these agents results in a percentage of patients having an improvement that is better than the natural course of disease, then the number of patients required to conduct a study with suffi-cient power to resolve the treatment effect is high. One trial was designed to detect a 30% improvement in hearing with 90% power. The investigators concluded that 127 patients would be required for the study. Despite recruit-ing 45 clinical sites for the study and conducting the study over a 32-month period, the number of patients enrolled fell short of the goal. It seems reason-able to postulate that oral antiviral agents may have a beneficial effect that is difficult to prove experimentally without a large sample size. As an analogy, consider that the use of oral antiviral agents in the treatment of Bell's palsy was not supported in initial randomized placebo-controlled trials but was re-cently supported in a trial involving a large number of patients [55]. Gener-ally, for healthy patients, a short course of oral antiviral agents presents minimal risk and potential benefit, although the benefits have yet to be proved in clinical trials.

Hyperbaric oxygen

The use of hyperbaric oxygen therapy in the treatment of SHL dates back to at least 1979 [56]. Although little appears in the literature for much of the 1980s and early 1990s, there seems to be renewed interest in this treatment modality, with several reports in the past 10 years. Most of this literature comes from centers in Europe [37,57,58], with relatively few studies from the United States [59], suggesting a geographic difference in the application of this treatment. From a Cochrane database review, it was concluded that in certain patients, the application of hyperbaric oxygen therapy signifi-cantly improved hearing loss, but the clinical significance of the level of improvement is not clear [60]. In their review of the literature, Conlin and Parnes [41,42] concluded that no valid randomized controlled trial exists to determine effective treatment of SHL, including hyperbaric oxygen treatment.

Practical management

The lack of suitable scientific data to base treatment regimens on leaves the clinician in an undesirable position when faced with a patient who has SHL. In most instances, the treatment is patient specific, with the goal of maximizing benefit and minimizing risk: more aggressive treatment is offered to those who have more severe losses, those whose hearing loss may present substantial lifestyle impact or employment difficulties (eg, professional musicians), and those who do not have other medical conditions that might be worsened by potential treatment agents (eg, normal renal and hepatic function and the absence of diabetes). In 1996, Hughes and colleagues [4] provided a respected and useful review of this topic, which concluded by suggesting how the senior investigator might treat himself if he were to have SHL. The current authors present here their current protocol for treatment of SHL and how the senior author might treat himself were he to suffer SHL: the evaluation would include a history and physical examination as described earlier, contrast-enhanced MRI, and complete audiometry. Treatment would begin with a prednisone oral taper, starting at 60 mg daily, tapered over 2 weeks, along with concurrent administration of an oral antiviral agent, given for 1 week. If no objective improvement had been obtained after completion of medical therapy, then a transtympanic dexamethasone perfusion would be offered as salvage therapy. If presentation for treatment had been delayed, oral steroid therapy would potentially be offered up to 6 weeks from the onset of symptoms. Transtympanic steroids could also potentially be employed up to 6 weeks from the onset of symptoms. Although 6 weeks may seem late, it is not uncommon to have a patient present to the clinic in this time frame without having received systemic or transtympanic steroids. Although the authors would treat a previously untreated patient for up to 6 weeks, patients who receive a short or inadequate course of steroids early in the course of the disease are generally not re-treated with a more standard course of steroids when seen after 2 to 3 weeks. Carbogen inhalation, vasodilators, and other previously described therapies are not currently offered.

Summary

SHL remains one of the more interesting and disputed topics in otolaryngology. It is a topic of seemingly boundless discussion and active research. In most cases, SHL is the presenting symptom of an emergency for which we have yet to find a convincing cause or reliable treatment. Treatment varies dramatically among practitioners and regions; however, in the United States, many practitioners generally consider offering a course of oral steroids for patients in whom no other contradictory medical condition exists. The use of other treatments has been well described and should be carefully considered. Ongoing large-scale research projects may soon provide a greater understanding of how to more optimally manage SHL.

References

[1] Mattox DE, Lyles CA. Idiopathic sudden sensorineural hearing loss. Am J Otol 1989;10(3): 242–3.
[2] Fetterman BL, Saunders JE, Luxford WM. Prognosis and treatment of sudden sensorineural hearing loss. Am J Otol 1996;17:529–36.

[3] Mattox DE, Simmons FB. Natural history of sudden sensorineural hearing loss. Ann Otol Rhinol Laryngol 1977;86:463–80.

[4] Hughes GB, Freedman MA, Haberkamp TJ, et al. Sudden sensorineural hearing loss. Otolaryngol Clin North Am 1996;29:393–405.

[5] Cole RR, Jahrsdoerfer RA. Sudden hearing loss: an update. Am J Otol 1988;19(3): 211–5.

[6] Haberkamp TJ, Tanyeri HM. Management of idiopathic sudden sensorineural hearing loss. Am J Otol 1999;20:587–95.

[7] Byl FM Jr. Sudden hearing loss: eight years' experience and suggested prognostic table. Laryngoscope 1984;94:647–61.

[8] National Institute on Deafness and Other Communication Disorders (NIDCD). Sudden deafness. Available at: http://www.nidcd.nih.gov/health/hearing/sudden.asp. Accessed March 13, 2008.

[9] The United States Census Bureau US and World Population Clocks. Available at: http:// www.census.gov/main/www/popclock.html. March 13, 2008.

[10] Wu CS, Lin HC, Chao PZ. Sudden sensorineural hearing loss: evidence from Taiwan. Audiol Neurootol 2006;11:151–6.

[11] Tran Ba Huey P, Sauvaget E. Idiopathic sudden sensorineural hearing loss is not an otologic emergency. Otol Neurotol 2005;26:896–902.

[12] Kakehata S, Sasaki A, Oji K, et al. Comparison of intratympanic and intravenous dexamethasone treatment on sudden sensorineural hearing loss with diabetes. Otol Neurotol 2006;27: 604–8.

[13] Choung YH, Park K, Shin YR, et al. Intratympanic dexamethasone injection for refractory sudden sensorineural hearing loss. Laryngoscope 2006;116:747–52.

[14] Dallan I, Bruschini L, Nacci A, et al. Transtympanic steroids as a salvage therapy in sudden hearing loss: preliminary results. ORL J Otorhinolaryngol Relat Spec 2006;68: 247–52.

[15] Wilson WR, Byl FM, Laird N. The efficacy of steroids in the treatment of idiopathic sudden hearing loss. A double-blind clinical study. Arch Otolaryngol 1980;106:772–6.

[16] Yeo SW, Lee DH, Jun BC, et al. Hearing outcome of sudden sensorineural hearing loss: long-term follow-up. Otolaryngol Head Neck Surg 2007;136:221–4.

[17] Wilkins SA, Mattox DE, Lyles A. Evaluation of a shotgun regimen for sudden hearing loss. Otolaryngol Head Neck Surg 1987;97:474–80.

[18] Haynes DS, O'Malley M, Cohen S, et al. Intratympanic dexamethasone for sudden sensorineural hearing loss after failure of systemic therapy. Laryngoscope 2007;117: 3–15.

[19] Lazarini PR, Camargo AC. Idiopathic sudden sensorineural hearing loss: etiopathogenic aspects. Rev Bras Otorrinolaringol (Engl Ed) 2006;72(4):554–61.

[20] Rybak LP. Treatable sensorineural hearing loss. Am J Otol 1985;6(6):482–9.

[21] Stokroos RJ, Albers FW, Schirm J. Therapy of idiopathic sudden sensorineural hearing loss: antiviral treatment of experimental herpes simplex virus infection of the inner ear. Ann Otol Rhinol Laryngol 1999;108:423–8.

[22] Cummins D, McCormick JB, Bennett D, et al. Acute sensorineural deafness in Lassa fever. JAMA 1990;264:2093–6.

[23] Liao BS, Byl FM, Adour KK. Audiometric comparison of Lassa fever hearing loss and idiopathic sudden hearing loss: evidence for viral cause. Otolaryngol Head Neck Surg 1992;106:226–9.

[24] Son EJ, Bang JH, Kang JG. Anterior inferior cerebellar artery infarction presenting with sudden hearing loss and vertigo. Laryngoscope 2007;117(3):556–8.

[25] Rudack C, Langer C, Stoll W, et al. Vascular risk factors in sudden hearing loss. Thromb Haemost 2006;95:454–61.

[26] Capaccio P, Ottaviani F, Cuccarini V, et al. Genetic and acquired prothrombotic risk factors and sudden hearing loss. Laryngoscope 2007;117:547–51.

[27] Finger RP, Gostian AO. Apheresis for idiopathic sudden hearing loss: reviewing the evidence. J Clin Apheresis 2006;21:241–5.

[28] McCabe BF. Autoimmune sensorineural hearing loss. Ann Otol Rhinol Laryngol 1979;88: 585–9.

[29] Harris JP, Sharp PA. Inner ear autoantibodies in patients with rapidly progressive sensorineural hearing loss. Laryngoscope 1990;100:516–24.

[30] Berrocal JR, Ramirez-Camacho R. Sudden sensorineural hearing loss: supporting the immunologic theory. Ann Otol Rhinol Laryngol 2002;111:989–97.

[31] Committee on Hearing and Equilibrium guidelines for the diagnosis and evaluation of therapy in Meniere's disease. Otolaryngol Head Neck Surg 1995;113(3):181–5.

[32] Lorenzi MC, Bittar RS, Pedalini ME, et al. Sudden deafness and Lyme disease. Laryngoscope 2003;113:312–5.

[33] Peltomaa M, Pyykko I, Seppala I, et al. Lyme borreliosis: an etiological factor in sensorineural hearing loss? Eur Arch Otorhinolaryngol 2000;257:317–22.

[34] Hughes GB, Rutherford I. Predictive value of serologic tests for syphilis in otology. Ann Otol Rhinol Laryngol 1986;(3 Pt 1):250–9.

[35] Klemm E, Bepperling F, Burschka MA, et al. Hemodilution therapy with hydroxyethyl starch solution (130/0.4) in unilateral idiopathic sudden sensorineural hearing loss: a dose-finding, double-blind, placebo-controlled, international multicenter trial with 210 patients. Otol Neurotol 2007;28(2):157–70.

[36] Slattery WH, Fisher LM, Iqbal Z, et al. Oral steroid regimens for idiopathic sudden sensorineural hearing loss. Otolaryngol Head Neck Surg 2005;132:5–10.

[37] Narozny W, Sicko Z, Przewozny T, et al. Usefulness of high doses of glucocorticoids and hyperbaric oxygen therapy in sudden sensorineural hearing loss treatment. Otol Neurotol 2004;25(6):916–23.

[38] Cinamon U, Bendet E, Kronenberg J. Steroids, carbogen or placebo for sudden hearing loss: a prospective double-blind study. Eur Arch Otorhinolaryngol 2001;258:477–80.

[39] Minoda R, Masuyama K, Habu K, et al. Initial steroid hormone dose in the treatment of idiopathic sudden deafness. Am J Otol 2000;21(6):819–25.

[40] Wei BP, Mubiru S, O'Leary S. Steroids for idiopathic sudden sensorineural hearing loss. Cochrane Database Syst Rev 2006;(1) CD003998.

[41] Conlin AE, Parnes LS. Treatment of sudden sensorineural hearing loss: I. A systematic review. Arch Otolaryngol Head Neck Surg 2007;133(6):573–81.

[42] Conlin AE, Parnes LS. Treatment of sudden sensorineural hearing loss: II. A meta-analysis. Arch Otolaryngol Head Neck Surg 2007;133(6):582–6.

[43] Itoh A, Sakata E. Treatment of vestibular disorders. Acta Otolaryngol Suppl 1991;481: 617–23.

[44] Silverstein H, Choo D, Rosenberg SI, et al. Intratympanic steroid treatment of inner ear disease and tinnitus (preliminary report). Ear Nose Throat J 1996;75:468–71.

[45] Parnes LS, Sun AH, Freeman DJ. Corticosteroid pharmacokinetics in the inner ear fluids: an animal study followed by clinical application. Laryngoscope 1999;109:1–17.

[46] Chandrasekhar SS. Intratympanic dexamethasone for sudden sensorineural hearing loss: clinical and laboratory evaluation. Otol Neurotol 2001;22:18–23.

[47] Gianoli GJ, Li JC. Transtympanic steroids for treatment of sudden hearing loss. Otolaryngol Head Neck Surg 2001;125:142–6.

[48] Gouveris H, Selivanova O, Mann W. Intratympanic dexamethasone with hyaluronic acid in the treatment of idiopathic sudden sensorineural hearing loss after failure of intravenous steroid and vasoactive therapy. Eur Arch Otorhinolaryngol 2005;262:131–4.

[49] Ho GM, Lin HG, Shu MT. Effectiveness of intratympanic dexamethasone injection in sudden deafness patients as salvage treatment. Laryngoscope 2004;114:1184–9.

[50] Herr BD, Marzo SJ. Intratympanic steroid perfusion for refractory sudden sensorineural hearing loss. Otolaryngol Head Neck Surg 2005;132:527–31.

[51] Kanemaru S, Fukushima H, Nakamura H, et al. Alpha-interferon for the treatment of idiopathic sudden sensorineural hearing loss. Eur Arch Otorhinolaryngol 1997;254(3): 158–62.

[52] Zadeh MH, Storper IS, Spitzer JB. Diagnosis and treatment of sudden-onset sensorineural hearing loss: a study of 51 patients. Otolaryngol Head Neck Surg 2003;128(1):92–8.

[53] Stokroos RJ, Albers FW, Tenvergert EM. Antiviral treatment of idiopathic sudden sensori-neural hearing loss: a prospective, randomized, double-blind clinical trial. Acta Otolaryngol 1998;118:488–95.

[54] Tucci DL, Farmer JC, Kitch RD, et al. Treatment of sudden sensorineural hearing loss with systemic steroids and acyclovir. Otol Neurotol 2002;23:301–8.

[55] Hato N, Yamada H, Kohno H, et al. Valacyclovir and prednisolone treatment for Bell's palsy: a multicenter, randomized, placebo-controlled study. Otol Neurotol 2007;28(3): 408–13.

[56] Goto F, Fujita T, Kitani Y, et al. Hyperbaric oxygen and stellate ganglion blocks for idiopathic sudden hearing loss. Acta Otolaryngol 1979;88(5–6):335–42.

[57] Narozny W, Kuczkowski J, Mikaszewski B. HBO effectively supports SSNHL therapy. Eur Arch Otorhinolaryngol 2005;262(2):163–4.

[58] Racic G, Maslovara S, Roje Z, et al. Hyperbaric oxygen in the treatment of sudden hearing loss. ORL J Otorhinolaryngol Relat Spec 2003;65(6):317–20.

[59] Horn CE, Himel HN, Selesnick SH. Hyperbaric oxygen therapy for sudden sensorineural hearing loss: a prospective trial of patients failing steroid and antiviral treatment. Otol Neurotol 2005;26(5):882–9.

[60] Bennett MH, Kertesz T, Yeung P. Hyperbaric oxygen for idiopathic sudden sensorineural hearing loss and tinnitus. Cochrane Database Syst Rev 2007;1:CD004739.

ELSEVIER
SAUNDERS

Otolaryngol Clin N Am
41 (2008) 651–655

OTOLARYNGOLOGIC
CLINICS
OF NORTH AMERICA

Index

Note: Page numbers of article titles are in **boldface** type.

A

Abscess. See specific types/locations of abscess.

Aerodigestive tract, upper, foreign bodies in, diagnosis and management of, **485–496**

Airway, difficult, **567–580**
  adults with, 569
  children with, 569
  definition of, 567
  equipment needed for, 572
  evaluation of, 568–572
  imaging studies in, 571
  management at level of obstruction, 577
  management of, 572–577
  securing for general anesthesia, 573–575
  surgical interventions in, 575–577
  urgent, 571–572
  impairment of, differential diagnosis of, 570

Airway management, in deep neck infections, 472–474

Amphotericin B, in invasive fungal sinusitis, 500

Antibiotics, and deep neck infections, 459

Antiviral agents, oral, in sudden hearing loss, 644–645

Artery, anterior ethmoid, anatomy of orbit and, 589–591
  splenopalatine, transnasal endoscopic ligation of, in epistaxis, 533–535

Aspiration pneumonia, in deep neck infection, 479

Atelectasis, in foreign bodies of upper aerodigestive tract, 488

Auricular nerve, great, as graft, in facial nerve paralysis, 627–628

B

Balloon catheter extraction, of esophageal foreign bodies, 494

Bell's palsy, as cause of facial paralysis, 620–621

Bleeding, orbital. See *Orbital hematoma.*

Blood vessels, injury to, in temporal bone fracture, 608

Bone fracture, temporal. See *Temporal bone fracture.*

Bronchoscope, flexible, intubation over, in difficult airway, 574

Buccal space, 467
  infections of, 467

C

Carotid sheath, 462–463

Carotid space, 469–470
  infections of, 470

Cavernous sinus thrombosis, as complication of rhinosinusitis, 512–513

Cellulitis, orbital, as complication of rhinosinusitis, 507–508
  preseptal, as complication of rhinosinusitis, 506–507

Cerebrospinal fluid leak(s), and orbital hematoma, during endoscopic sinus surgery, **581–596**
  ethmoid/cribiform, management of, 586–588
  frontal sinus, management of, 588–589
  in temporal bone fracture, 606, 611, 615
  intraoperative, 581–589
    management of, 584–586
  sphenoid sinus, management of, 588

Cervical fascia, of neck, 459, 460–463

doi:10.1016/S0030-6665(08)00063-7